W0227434

Mantras for Positive Ageing

Mantras for Positive Ageing

from 50 eminent Indians

WITH A FOREWORD BY
H. H. THE DALAI LAMA

EDITED BY
DR. V. MOHINI GIRI
MEERA KHANNA

Pippa Rann
books & media

Pippa Rann
books & media

An imprint of
Salt Desert Media Group Limited,
7 Mulgrave Chambers, 26 Mulgrave Rd,
Sutton SM2 6LE, England, UK.
Email: pubisher@pipparannbooks.com
Website: www.pipparannbooks.com

Copyright of the individual chapters belongs to the respective authors.
Copyright of the collection © Dr. V. Mohini Giri, Meera Khanna 2021.

All royalties from the sale of this book are dedicated to The Guild of Service.

The moral right of the authors and editors has been asserted.

The views and opinions expressed in this book are the authors' own and the facts are as reported by them, which have been verified to the extent possible, but the publishers are not in any way liable for the same.

All rights reserved. No part of this book may be reproduced by any mechanical, photographic, or electronic process, or in the form of a phonographic recording; nor may it be stored in a retrieval system, transmitted or otherwise be copied for public or private use – other than for 'fair use' as brief quotations embodied in articles and reviews, without prior written permission of the publisher.

ISBN 978-19-13738-51-8

Designed and typeset by Raghav Khattar

Printed and bound at Replika Press, Sonipat

FSC www.fsc.org MIX Paper from responsible sources FSC® C016779

Published on the occasion of
the Golden Jubilee of The Guild of Service

Contents

THE DALAI LAMA

FOREWORD

I am pleased that the Guild of Service (INDIA) has compiled this book on the art of ageing positively. Life has a beginning and in due course, an end. The important thing is for each of us to live our lives meaningfully and refrain from causing harm to others.

The most effective way to make meaningful use of the opportunity our lives offer us is to develop our concern for others. It is important to care for our physical health, however we must take particular care of our emotional hygiene. We must cultivate restraint from indulging in disturbing emotions such as anger, jealousy and craving in order to avoid the problems they cause. Such emotional training will also help us become more patient when we confront the challenges that naturally accompany aging.

Most importantly, I believe in the benefits of developing love and compassion towards others. When we were young, we were lovingly cared for by our parents. All of you in turn have cared for your family members, friends and colleagues with concern and affection. As a result of your kindness towards them, I am sure you are now able to enjoy their loving care.

I also deeply appreciate your Organisation's contribution towards uplifting the life of less privileged members of our society, especially women.

Several of the contributors to this book who have shared their thoughts and experiences about ageing, are friends I have known over the years. We have grown old together. I hope that readers will enjoy their insights and benefit from their positive outlook.

5 November 2020

PROLOGUE

This volume is a collection of articles from my gracious sisters and brothers on the occasion of the 50th year of the Guild's journey towards women's empowerment and social justice.

Befittingly there are 50 articles from people from all walks of life celebrities, eminent doctors, acclaimed artists, renowned lawyers, and impactful social activists. But there is one common denominator. All the writers have been in search of change and today we celebrate their strength. Their strength in contributing immensely to society and which has helped them to prove that age is only a number. This anthology reverberates with the message that the sky is the limit and big canvas of the earth is their playground.

The story of the journey of the Guild of Service can be traced back in 1971 when we realized that women in the patriarchal atmosphere were not only stifled but these unequal terms killed them. Our work has mapped changes in gender inequality in different sectors. Many of the contributors to this book have been agents of the quantum and direction of change. The Guild is a national level voluntary organization in consultative status with ECOSOC of the United Nations. The Guild does not work on the welfare model of developmental work but on the rights-based approach to build social, educational, economic, legal, and political capacities so that women are accorded the dignity that that are entitled to as citizens of this country.

Today the Guild runs three shelter homes in Vrindavan (for destitute widows), in Baramulla (for conflict affected women and children; now being transformed into a capacity building centre), and in Delhi (for working girls). The Guild successfully ran shelter homes in Godhra (for riot affected women), and in Tarangpadi and Nagapattinam (for tsunami-affected women), and closed them after the women were mainstreamed into normal lives post training for economic enhancement. The Guild also runs presently five capacity building centres in Vrindavan, Najafgarh, Jaipur, Sawai Madhopur, and Baramulla, where women are taught skills, where skill upgradation is facilitated, and where they are offered literacy skills to build their capacities to earn a decent livelihood. The Guild runs three schools for under privileged children, in Najafgarh (for children of migrant families), in Vrindavan (for children of the nearby villages), and in Jaipur (for slum children). The Guild also runs three Family Counselling Centres in Mathura, in Sawai Madhopur, and in Delhi, to provide counselling services and free legal aid to women from weaker sections of society who are victims of difficult circumstances. As part of its mandate of empowering women, the Guild has been conducting dowry-less ostentation-free mass-marriages since 1972. And conducting Interfaith Peace Prayers. With that wide experience, this volume questions the parameters normally used to measures changes in health, disorders, legal knowledge, nutrition, participation in work and how one can age gracefully with these parameters.

I would like to thank all the contributors to this volume who wrote not with the pen of nostalgia but with the laptop of productive ageing. Despite their various commitments they acceded to our request with alacrity.

My respectful pranaam and appreciation to Shree Shree His Holiness Dalai Lama ji for his kind Foreword. I would like to thank my dear friends for facilitating our connect to His Holiness The Dalai Lama.

I thank Dr. Mira Shiva for offering to translate Shri Sunderlal Bahuguna's handwritten Hindi essay into English.

I thank Renu and Sharla from the Guild secretariat for helping in the compilation of the contributions.

I would like to acknowledge with thanks our Executive Vice President Meera Khanna for editing the book.

Our motto is SERVE, LOVE, GIVE.

Dr. V. Mohini Giri

Section I
Age and Ageing: Facets and Facts

1
A Doctor in an Ageing Society
Dr. A. B. Dey

Disease, old age, and death are disturbing thoughts for the young and healthy since antiquity. As a physician, trained in learning the subject and in treating the young patient, this practitioner of modern medicine and teacher in academic institutions always felt greatly satisfied in unravelling the mysteries of complex symptoms (i.e., what a patient complains of) and signs (what a doctor elicits) and making an excellent diagnosis. The task is over once the diagnosis is made and then what happens to the patient and the family is not one's concern. Once the cause of an excruciating and unbearable pain is diagnosed it is the job of the anaesthetist or pain medicine specialist to relieve it. A disability is the responsibility of rehabilitation specialist. This arrangement suited one fine: to be considered as an intellectual and a problem solver, while the more intelligent organ specialist colleagues would be busy with their "stents and scopes". A quarter century back this comfortable professional life turned turtle for me as, in search of excitement, I started doing Geriatrics, or care of older persons, in which hardly anyone was interested at that time.

In last three decades, Geriatrics or Geriatric Medicine has evolved from an ill-defined entity of "internal medicine of older people" to a rapidly-growing distinct discipline which tries to unravel the biology behind the decaying and failing soma, and advise ways and means to preserve residual structure and function of organs – if not reverse the deficits that have accumulated over the years. Issues of ageing are better understood, and one has greater clarity about the biological progress. A famous biologist described ageing as the process that converts fit adults into frailer adults with a progressively increased risk of illness, injury, and death. Thus, geriatrics now is about intrinsic capacity, functional ability, and overcoming environmental challenges. For a young doctor it is a complex discipline.

In the last five years or so especially, the World Health Organization and scores of biologists and clinicians have changed the field. Geriatricians and gerontologists no longer feel apologetic about pleading the case of a group of human beings who have lived their lives and used to be considered fit to leave this world, leaving us to focus on other pressing issues of communicable diseases, heart disease, cancer, safe motherhood, and healthy childhood. If long life is the goal of disciplines of medicine, care of the long-living human beings logically becomes important. Ageing of individuals and societies is a global phenomenon resulting from declining fertility, improved survival during childhood, and progressive improvements in life expectancy over the past century. This trend is likely to continue well into the 21st century. Population ageing is a cause for celebration, representing the triumph of medical, social, and economic advances over disease and death. But the trend also presents tremendous challenges for the functioning of most institutions of society, including practice of medicine.

Ageing and age-related diseases have appeared as challenges facing health systems after satisfactory control over communicable diseases. The ageing process has a major causative association with a large number of diseases and disabilities due to biological decay and greater exposure to harmful risk factors. Medical education traditionally has been based on a "single disease" model. With overall increase in longevity globally, there is paradigm shift in understanding of diseases and their manifestations in clinical practice. It is important for physicians to gain a greater understanding of diseases of older persons and biological, social, and economic context that is associated with its causation and impact. Disease in older people is typically multi-factorial with a strong component of the underlying ageing process. Older people respond differently, and usually with more adverse reactions, to treatments and interventions than younger people. It is critical to appreciate the complete picture of an older person with multiple acute and chronic diseases and disabilities and poor functionality - and in an adverse psycho-social milieu - all of which will affect the health outcome. Patient who are old in age will account for one in every five persons by the middle of the twenty-first century. Today's medical student will soon be practising in a different clinical setting and thus needs to be prepared to face this new challenge for a successful and satisfying medical career.

The New Patient in Clinical Practice

We have a new patient in the clinic, the older patient. Pattern of diseases have shifted to non-communicable disease from communicable disease and this phenomenon invariably accompanies transition to an ageing society. In recent decades proportion of deaths due to infectious disease; and maternal and infant mortality, have fallen remarkably and non-communicable disease related deaths such as cardiovascular diseases, stroke, diabetes, cancer, and age-related neurodegenerative diseases have increased steadily. This shift reflects population ageing. One may enter old age in good health but, sooner or later, age itself turns into a risk factor for various non-communicable and communicable diseases.

Greater longevity provides a longer time window for the manifestation of exposure to known and unknown health risks and impact of biological decline in organ structure and function. Longer life also enhances the duration of exposure as well as biological decline. Consequently, older people carry a great burden of metabolic-vascular diseases; degenerative diseases of the brain, musculoskeletal system, and sensory organs; cancer;

chronic lung disease; and greater risk of infectious diseases. These age-related diseases also lead to various disabilities and decline in the overall functional capacity of the older person. The large burden of disease and functional decline requires easy and rapid access to quality primary and specialist health services, adequate financial resources and caregiver support for nursing and assistance in activities of daily living. A composite description of the health status of older patients would be multi-morbidity, multiple disabilities, poor functionality, and lack of resources to access health care.

Impact on Society and Family

Population ageing is poised to become one of the most significant social transformations of the twenty-first century, with implications for several institutions of the society; namely: family, community, health system, social welfare system; and pension and financial services. The benefits of greater longevity to individuals, families, and society can be manifold. Longer lives can afford individuals opportunities to prolong their working life, embark on second careers, or pursue varied interests in old age. Families benefit from the contributions of older generations, for example, through financial support, assistance with household maintenance, or participation in childcare. Societies benefit from the wisdom and experience of older persons and from their contributions to the labour force, as well as from their volunteerism, philanthropy, and civic engagement. At the same time, many are concerned about the implications of population ageing, as the need for socio-economic support increases for the older population. Moreover, population ageing and growth in the number of persons at very advanced ages put pressure on health systems, which must adapt to meet the growing demand for care, services, and technologies to prevent and treat non-communicable diseases and chronic conditions associated with old age.

Care of Older Persons at Home and Institutions

Older Indians prefer to live and age at the place where they have spent most of their lives. It has been a common observation in clinical practice that older people prefer to die in their homes rather than in hospital or hospice. While health services are available in public health or private health services, the care of the elderly is a responsibility of the family. At some point in time, almost every individual, especially in old age, would lose his or her ability to survive independently due to limited mobility, frailty, the decline in physical health due to various acute or chronic disease or dementia. With the loss of autonomy, the individual is dependent on others for pursuing basic activities of daily living and may require assistance from some form of long- term care.

Community based surveys have shown that nearly a quarter of people above the age of 80 years are home bound or bed bound, while the proportion is about 7% of all who are above 60 years of age. Extrapolating these numbers to current population one arrives at a figure of 8 to 10 million Indians, who are home or bed bound. While homebound persons are likely to be disabled with locomotor or visual disability, bed-bound persons are most likely to be completely or partially dependent on caregivers, with different grades of care requirement. A homebound person requires assistance in instrumental activities of daily living (IADL) while a bed bound person requires assistance in basic activities of daily living (BADL). In either case, these individuals are in need of assistance and care from family members and formal caregivers.

Long-term care of the bed-bound patient, who may have dementia or stroke or sheer frailty, is a challenging task in view of the variable length and quantity of such care. Three issues are of great importance in long-term care:

- assistance in activities of daily living, especially personal hygiene;
- treatment of chronic diseases and disabilities; and
- acute health problems which are often unanticipated and disturb the stability of the care arrangements.

Institutional long-term care is virtually non-existent in India due to cultural and economic factors. In Indian society, inter-generational relationships, caring, ill health, etc. are considered private issues and generally kept within the confines of the family. The family with or without paid help would provide the physical care whereas the local general practitioner is the main source of medical care at the community level.

The issues related to long-term care need in the Indian context are diverse. The quantum of care depends on whether the patient is cognitively intact or not. Dementia patients need greater volume of care, and are more difficult to manage. Both public and private hospitals, being acute care set-ups with pressure on bed availability, do not participate in long-term care. Old age homes do a detailed health assessment before admitting older persons. In the event of the individual suffering from a major health problem and losing independence, many of these homes would force the next of kin to withdraw the family member, while charitable homes would continue to care. Hospices are available in India but mostly for cancer patients with very few takers. Rarely does an institution admit dependent person requiring minimal medical care and maximal nursing care for an unforeseen period of time, except charitable organisations and hospices that too only those persons who are likely to die in foreseeable future. Day care services are very few and there are very few takers for such services. There is no financial mechanism for supporting long-term care in India. Old-age homes without any health infrastructure are alternatives for accommodation for those older persons who lack shelter or cannot stay with family. There are less than 50,000 old-age home beds in India. There are three types of management of old-age homes: charity, for-profit, and public sector. The old-age home industry is mostly unregulated with no defined minimum standards.

Many Diseases Together that Manifest Unusually

One of the greatest challenges in geriatric medicine is the optimal management of older adults with multiple chronic conditions, or "multi-morbidity"; which is defined as presence of two or more diseases together at any point of time. Complex problems with simple solutions do not exist for older patients. Multiple complaints and abnormal findings will always arise from multiple diseases; discovering a diagnosis that unifies all the symptoms, signs and laboratory abnormalities is rare. It is important to remember that patients can have a multiplicity of diseases.

Multi-morbidity prevalence increases with age, and can be as high as 90% in community-dwelling older adults aged 75 years and above. Multi-morbidity is associated with many adverse consequences: disability, need for repeated hospitalisation, poor functional status, poor quality of life, need for multiple medications and higher rates of complications from illnesses, risk of adverse reaction from drugs and interventions; and risk of death. Not many practice guidelines exist for multi-morbidity in older patients as trials and guidelines nearly always focus on the management of a single disease in younger patients. Older adults with multi-morbidity are heterogeneous in terms of severity of illness, functional status, prognosis, personal priorities, and risk of adverse events even when diagnosed with the same pattern of conditions. Thus, a single solution with "one size fits all" is not practical and one needs to have a flexible approach to care in these patients.

Older patients with many diseases usually present themselves with atypical symptoms. Blunting, or absence of typical or classical signs and symptoms, is well recorded for many conditions. A patient with pneumonia may come with the symptom only of altered senses, a patient with myocardial infarction may come exclusively with recurrent episodes of vomiting, or a patient with urinary tract infection because of a fall. The literature divides atypical presentations into three main categories: vague or non-specific symptoms; unusual or altered symptoms from what is normally expected; and lack of symptoms.

Failure to recognize atypical presentations may lead to worse outcomes, missed diagnoses, and missed opportunities for treatment of common conditions in older patients. Non-specific presentations may include more than one non-specific geriatric syndromes (e.g., delirium, fall, incontinence, fatigue, functional decline, syncope, dizziness, weight loss). The likely explanation is that interactions between biological ageing and chronic diseases restrict the capacity to maintain homeostasis and any perturbation by disease manifests in the most vulnerable organ or weakest link. The lesson here for the physician is that when faced with such a presentation, a comprehensive evaluation is the only appropriate clinical response. Underreporting of symptoms is also a common behaviour among elderly with dangerous consequences. Many symptoms are considered part of normal ageing by both the patient and family, sometimes perpetuated by clinicians who often have an image of older patients - with infinite complaints whose investigation lead nowhere. Late recognition leads to delayed intervention, usually after substantial morbidity associated with advanced pathology has already ensued with major functional losses.

Conclusion

The population boom is real and the challenge of caring for older population is huge. Geriatric Medicine is one of the most complex specialties in medicine. Older patients invariably harbour one or more non-communicable diseases along with mental health problems and carry a large burden of disabilities and decay in sensory organ often due to irreversible biological decline. In the very old and bed/bound, maladies are present in multiples, affecting functional status, health service requirements, health care expenditure, and drug consumption. A holistic multidisciplinary approach at an individual level is needed to address these issues. A single and simple change can have a huge impact in the health of older adults.

2
THE DESTITUTION OF AGEING WIDOWHOOD

MATHEW CHERIAN

"I am uncompromising in the matter of women's rights. In my opinion she should labour under no legal disability, not suffered by man. I should treat daughters and sons on a footing of perfect equality."

– Mahatma Gandhi

In the last months of 2017, HelpAge India was suddenly summoned by the Court based on a Public Interest Litigation (PIL) to look after widows in Vrindavan, Mathura, by an order of the Supreme Court looking at their depressing situation, deep poverty, and exploitation, in one of the holiest cities of India, the birthplace of Lord Krishna who is the succour of millions across India. Even in the holiest of places, widows do not find any relief for their existence on earth. The plight of these widows is one area that has not been solved in our seventy odd years of the independent republic, which should have been a priority.

Raja Ram Mohan Roy campaigned, with the support of Ishwar Chandra Vidyasagar, for widow remarriage in undivided Bengal, and Lord Bentinck promulgated an ordinance to promote widow remarriage called the Hindu Widow Remarriage Act of 1856. But older women, especially widows, are still unwelcome in many families due to stigma associated to them by the Hindu religion. In some cases, their heads are shaved, and they are forced to wear a white saree with no bangles or bindi. This could not be better designed to completely destroy the self-esteem of a woman who is already in a trauma because of her husband's death. Some blame particularly the Vaishnavite tradition for such oppression. But another factor is the economic burden that an unproductive and expensive older woman brings to the family due to medical care. Very often she is not treated for poor health and the women themselves do not express their health problems out of fear and ignorance. The burden is heaviest in the case of poor and destitute families. Even today there are 22 million Indian widows who have no reliable means of sustenance – in other words, no Widow Pension or social security. Though there is a Widow Pension given by Government of India, that covers only 1.2 million women - just about 5% of the widow population in India. And that Pension from the Government is a meagre 200 rupees per month. HelpAge India has recommended a universal pension of 2000 rupees per month to all widows considering the triple burden they face in society. Even the Lord does not protect the poor widow in Krishna Janmabhoomi and they need some social security from the state. After a century and a half, we have still not eliminated the problems of widows in old age. Widow pensions do not reach them. The state of pensions is a very vexed issue in India.

The National Old Age Pension scheme (NOAPS) under the National Social Assistance Programme (NSAP), was introduced as a Centrally Sponsored Scheme in the year 1995. At that time, the scheme provided a monthly pension of Rs 75 to a destitute older person over the age of 65. The limited coverage of the scheme was basically due to resource constraints. Only 5 million, out of the 8.71 million eligible beneficiaries, were covered under the scheme using funds from the Central Government. On 1 April 2000, a new scheme called Annapurna was launched with the objective of providing food security to the destitute that were not being covered under the National Old Age Pension Scheme. This scheme was expected to cover 20% of the older persons eligible for NOAPS. The scheme was not received well by the States: some refused to implement it, and others demanded modifications. In the year 2001–2, as against the target of 1.34 million persons, only 15% could be covered.

In 2007, NOAPS was renamed as Indira Gandhi National Old Age Pension Scheme (IGNOAPS) along with Widow Pensions and made applicable to all older persons belonging to families living below the poverty line called the National Social Assistance Programme. The central contribution per beneficiary per month was increased to Rs 200. In the year 2011, the age criterion was reduced to 60 years and the monthly amount was increased to Rs 500 for older persons of age 80 and above. In the year 2002–3, the scheme covered 7.4 million older people and in the year 2010–11, this number was 17 million. In addition, 0.8 million were covered under Annapurna (a food scheme for below poverty line people) in the year 2002–3; the number went up to1 million in the year 2010–11. The inadequacy of the provision, both in terms of the number of beneficiaries, and in terms of the amount provided, should be seen in the context of the rise in the cost of living over the years, and lack of a properly integrated and national health care system.

Many widows in Vrindavan are yet to be covered under the Right to Food. Without a formal identity or an UID card they are still not under the ambit of any Public Distribution System. They spend the whole day singing bhajans in the temples and receive few rupees and a little bit of "prasad" (a small offering from the god which is usually sweet). Many widows are diabetic and do not have any form of treatment. HelpAge India's medical vans have been treating them and offering medical help, thanks to a single donor (Mrs Chuttani) who has donated the entire funding to help these widows after seeing their plight. The widows have also become a bone of contention between Governments of Uttar Pradesh and West Bengal. There have been constant intergovernmental letters to take back the widows to Bengal. Another organization, Akshay Patra, has offered cooked food to many of the widows. However, many widows have complained that they prefer rice, while it is *chappathis* that are offered by the NGO. It is also quite ridiculous that Government of Uttar Pradesh wrote to Government of West Bengal to take these widows back. However, after much lobbying many widows were able to get their UID card in early 2014.

Many older widows suffer from depression and need treatment. According to Dr. Prof A. B. Dey head of geriatric medicine at AIIMS, "older women are more prone to depression and their mental health is rarely attended to "and in the case of Vrindavan widows it is far worse. The case in Vrindavan homes is more to highlight the problems that face older women in India every day. It is almost a truism that older women would be discriminated in the patriarchal society of South Asia. Many in India feel that in a traditional society, social change is necessary if women are to be given respect, care and dignity. There were social systems that guaranteed respect as well as security for the aged. The modern economy with technological advancement makes the traditional knowhow of the elderly somewhat redundant be it oral history or folktales, or even the application of traditional remedies which grandmothers used to give to children.

I came across work in relation to the needs of widows through Mrs Mohini Giri and the Guild of Service, and their commendable work in fact in many spheres. In the summer of 2010, we began working on the draft of the National Policy on Ageing. This committee was chaired by Dr. Mohini Giri and some of my learnings came from her wide experience of older women and their fundamental issues. We are able to document the extent of their suffering, and the discrimination they faced in their home villages, and with their families. No wonder many fled to Vrindavan, the abode of Lord Krishna.

Elderly Women and Single Women Need More Help than Older Men

The oldest of elderly women (i.e., over the age of 80) constitute an especially vulnerable group. An overwhelming proportion of this group are widows who in India suffer multiple misery – being women, being widows, being poor, and having longer agonising years to live than men. The phenomenon of ageing of the 80+ with enormous load of multiple morbidities needs urgent attention and consideration. This group suffers more on account of disability, chronic disease, terminal illness, dementia and depression, accidents, falls, nutritional deficiencies, loneliness etc. Some of these diseases have no cure as yet. Further, this group is subject to elderly abuse, as neglect and isolation which make them financially and emotionally dependent on families and others. It is important to make the 80+ financially self-sustaining. Their pension needs to be improved and there should be provision for free medical aid particularly for those who are exempt from paying Income Tax. They constitute only about 1% of the total population of India and in absolute number this is currently around 10 million, though it is expected to grow to around 53 million by the year 2050 – i.e., 3.5% of total population.

When we garnered this information, Mrs Giri constituted a special committee to look at the issues facing older women. When the committee gave its report, they highlighted the following issues.

Suggesting Policy Change with a Gender Perspective

The goal of a National Policy of Older Persons (NPOP) should be to have a gender perspective at all levels including planning, programming, budgeting, maintenance, and evaluation. The policy should be widely discussed to encourage appropriate responses. The Policy need to:

- Create an enabling environment through positive social and economic policies for older men and women to realize their full potential

- Provide access to health care, and economic, financial, and social security for older men and women, whether in rural or in urban areas
- Make a comprehensive and uniform pension scheme which includes widows by putting in place practices that are user-friendly, keeping ground realities in mind
- Strengthen legal systems for eliminating all forms of age discrimination, violence and abuse of older men and women
- Encourage change in social attitudes and community practices for active participation and involvement of older men and women in national development.

Older people, particularly women who are illiterate or oppressed, should be provided legal literacy and support to access their rights. The struggle to get older women their rights still continues. The Supreme Court's intervention, referred to at the start of this chapter, suggested several long-term measures, including:

- Identification of vulnerable women, and pro-active outreach to them
- Protection from domestic violence
- Access to social security schemes
- Access to affordable health interventions
- Availability of livelihood and financial support
- Financial literacy and empowerment
- Protection of property
- Focus on prevention of child marriage and thus early widowhood
- Focus on promotion of community-based single-women networks and housing

The effort to implement these has been led by Dr. Giri, and we hope that her efforts, along with those of others, can soon achieve some minimum care for those who are suffering the destitution of ageing widowhood.

3
Successful Ageing: Keeping an Active and Involved Mind
Dr. Mala Kapur Shankardass

I write this chapter on the basis of my own experience of ageing, as well as my academic research and my activist work with older people. I adopt a social science and public health perspective rather than the purely medical one which has dominated the discussions on ageing and mind since a long time.

Ageing is a very variable phenomenon. How we grow old is a personal choice, within the bounds set by the environment and by circumstances. Today, we have forty year-olds looking and feeling like an old person, but there are also older folks going back to education in their 50s, starting businesses in their 60s, training for triathlons in their 70s and, yes, having sex in their 80s, forgetting all about the tradition of renouncing the world and adopting the traditional ideal of a *vanprasth* lifestyle in later years. Positive and healthy attitude to ageing goes with longevity: researchers have found that negative stereotypes about ageing can actually shorten life. A Yale University study done few years back and quoted in the *Journal of Personality and Social Psychology* found that people who have a positive perception of ageing tend to live seven and a half years longer than those who don't. The difference may be the result of a better response to stress or even just the will to live, as reported in the study.

Many other studies indicate that the presence of social support makes both men and women less vulnerable to health problems. Research also suggests that widowhood adds to the risk of health problems and those in the ages 50 to 90 who describe themselves as lonely are particularly at risk. Some observations from my work on older people reveals that loneliness and isolation caused by death of a spouse is a precipitating factor for early death of the partner left behind. Studies conducted abroad suggest that isolated older people have death rates 2-4 times higher than those with strong social ties. As quoted by doctors and older people themselves, "It's really important to have confidantes and social support for general health. We all need something to look forward to that will get us up in the morning."

As the older population is increasing, more positive attitudes on old age are developing. Today the aged view themselves more positively because they are generally better educated, financially more secure, and in better health than their parents. A large majority of older people contribute effectively to society. Many are employed and work regularly. It is a myth that older people are unproductive and mainly sad and lonely. In our country only about 5% of people over 65 live in institutions. While it is true that demand for old age homes is increasing, the reason for that is not only neglect. The increase in demand is also associated with increasing nuclearization of families, migration – and desire for independence by older people themselves. A study in pay-and-stay homes with appropriate facilities and amenities, conducted by my non-government organization, Development, Welfare and Research Foundation (DWRF), revealed that only 15% of older people are lonely and unhappy among the 675 older people who reported their self-perceptions. And, for many of those, it is a problem which can be overcome with participation in community or with voluntary work and by consciously developing hobbies, a circle of friends and keeping their minds active.

So far as the function of the intellect is concerned, medical opinion again and again states that there is no reason to believe in the reduction of the function of the brain and mind as age advances unless there is presence of actual disease affecting them. We as social scientists and the medical community often make the mistake of comparing older persons with the young contemporaries exposed to a different social and technological world. Undeniably, there is some decline in physical strength in old age, and there are usually age-related deficiencies in the functioning of some of the organs, particularly the sense organs, the ears and the eyes. However, studies comparing the young with older people unaffected by age-related diseases such as dementia, Parkinson, or hypertension, indicates that mental functioning of people declines much less in later years than was supposed. Many old people, who happen to have maintained, throughout life, an active interest in any subject, including technology and its application, are found to perform well above average even when compared with young people.

In other words, growing older does not mean that mental abilities will necessarily be reduced. There's a lot that people can do to keep their mind sharp and alert. Researchers believe that many of the supposed age-related changes that affect the mind, such as memory loss, are actually lifestyle related. Just as muscles get flabby from sitting around and doing nothing, so does the brain. If regular workouts are not given to the brain, its functions will decline. Researchers from across the world have found that memory loss can be improved by 30 to 50 per cent simply by doing mental exercises. However, in some older people a marked decline in mental abilities may be due to factors like prescription medications or disease. Older people are more likely to take a range of medications for chronic conditions than younger people. It is true that good nutrition helps to keep the brain in optimum condition but adopting a more social science perspective I would like to discuss some social activities which contribute to improving mental fitness.

Keeping a reasonably active social life and engaging in plenty of stimulating activities and conversations does lead to better adjusted and happier old age. Older women involved with household activities have less psychological problems than those without work and those retired older men who have not come to term with their 'non-working' life. In this context I would like to promote the possibility of day care centres and of recreation outlets for older people, and their involvement with reading and thinking activities. Developing a hobby or an interest in later years contributes significantly to wellbeing. It is also now being advocated that involvement with activities which challenge the intellect and memory bring down the risk of dementia, Alzheimer's, and related disorders. It is observed that playing chess, cards, watching 'question and answer' game shows on television can improve the brain's functioning and awareness of people at any age. Also, it is believed that there are ways to improve a failing memory no matter what your age. Good recall is a learned skill and studies on older people indicate that paying attention to whatever it is they want to remember does work. In fact, much of our folklore on older people recognizes this fact. My work with older people has shown that using memory triggers, like association or visualization techniques, can reduce problems of memory loss. If older people, like those much younger, are busy thinking about something else, they will forget where they have put the house keys. Stress can cause memory lapses. Keeping stress under control with meditation and regular relaxation can contribute to coping better with life. Laughter clubs, mediation groups, participation in *satsangs* all have a positive role to play in the life of the individuals as much as the practice of using memory.

Without going into the medical causes and terminology, I would like to state that some of the conditions that can affect the brain's ability to function, such as stroke, are associated with diet, obesity, and sedentary lifestyle choices. Keeping an active body is crucial for an active mind. As a public policy for an ageing society, it becomes crucial to emphasise the importance of physical activity. There is ample research to suggest that regular exercise can improve memory, reasoning abilities, and reaction times. Public health messages for active and successful ageing in society must incorporate the value of 30 minutes of moderate exercise every day not only to deliver an oxygen boost to the brain but also to deliver significant other health benefits.

The benefits of positive thinking are many. Keeping lives happy and harmonious in old age can often be difficult but studies have shown that positive thinking can help to deal more effectively with everyday stress as well as having a beneficial effect on the emotional health. Research has also demonstrated that a persons' emotional well-being plays an important part in his or her physical health. It can be enormously beneficial, psychologically and physically, to make an effort to integrate positive thinking into every aspect of life. It is often much easier to be negative and critical, so an effort should be made to be positive and encouraging to yourself and to others. It is better to view crises as problems that can be solved. Focusing on good things in life helps to lessen stress. When faced with stressful situations, indulging in calming strategies such as taking deep breaths or visualizing tranquil scenes or images is useful. Depression is experienced by the older population, but is under-diagnosed and under-treated, and it needs proper attention.

The most important factor in successful later years is remaining intellectually, socially, and physically engaged with life. To do this, especially when the rhythms of the work-related world are terminated, is to figure out new things with which to be involved.

As the world's population of older people is increasing rapidly, we need to applaud the growing brigade of seniors who are socially connected, highly involved, and committed to projects and causes, open to new experiences, engaged in harbouring their strengths, applying their emotional maturity, and utilizing their regenerative capacities to grow and thrive in later years. We need to think together creatively to come up with imaginative and worthwhile ways of celebrating ageing.

Section II
Grace of Ageing

1
THE MANY DIMENSIONS OF AGEING
DR. KARAN SINGH

There are two things that we do from the moment that we are born all the way to the moment when we die, breathing and ageing. It is, therefore, necessary for us to be aware of the many methods of breathing which include pranayam and other such practices, as well as of the many dimensions of ageing. In this article I will deal only with ageing. I have identified five dimensions of ageing which are usually lumped together so that we can get a clear understanding of the various situations involved.

The first dimension is, of course, chronological depending on the date on which we are born. This can obviously not be legally changed, although it is often sought to be manipulated for admission to educational institutions! **Chronological age** being what it is, and our age expectancy steadily rising, it is important that the Central and State Governments should consider raising the age of retirement, where necessary. Special legal provisions also need to be made for the welfare of senior citizens, usually defined as those being over 60. There is the most unfortunate absence in India of suitable retirement homes where elderly people can spend their last years in comfort and dignity. These are at present few and far between and must be supplemented by special support from the Central and State Governments as well as NGOs & civil society.

Also, people retiring at 60 still have the capacity to contribute to society. This should be kept in mind by PSUs & NGOs where such people can be usefully employed, and advantage taken of their experience. Resident Welfare Associations can also involve retired people in various health and environment-related projects.

Physiological age is the second dimension. Some people are healthy at 80 and others unhealthy at 40. This depends considerably on the individual lifestyle adopted when we were young, including food habits (overeating is to be avoided), tobacco (smoking is an anti-social act because it poisons not only the smoker but all those all around), alcohol and drugs (these are highly addictive and cause severe psychosomatic damage), and a sedentary lifestyle (exercise remains essential for our whole life). This is where ancient disciplines such as yoga and taichi are of tremendous benefit. In other words what our health is when we become senior citizens will depend a great deal upon of the sort of lifestyle we have adopted when we were young, and of course on genetic factors beyond our control. Young people should, therefore, always remember that what they do when young will have a major impact on the quality of their later years.

The third dimension is **Emotional age**. Unfortunately, our educational system does not involve advice regarding how to maintain emotional stability. As a result of tension at the workplace and at home, and as we age, the loss of friends and dear ones, tension within the family, between husband and wife and between parents and children and financial problems all add up to the growing emotional trauma that we are now witnessing. There has been an exponential growth in mental illness and depression around the world with the pandemic and its dangers. This is particularly painful for elderly people and, therefore, we must through meditation, yoga or any other system learn to come to terms with our emotional problems. In India psychological counselling is still in its infancy and needs to be strengthened, although some gurus do fulfil this task. Trained counsellors can make a marked difference towards helping elderly people deal with their emotional problems.

The fourth dimension is **Intellectual age**. The body-mind relationships are now well established, and if we plan to have a healthy old age, our brain needs to function in a positive and creative manner. This involves the practice of reading, doing puzzles, playing indoor games and so on. We must always remember that the brain has an infinite capacity to grow. As a famous psychologist has said, "people do not grow old: when they stop growing, they become old". I have known people well into their 80s who remain sharp and creative. One such was the famous inventor of the geodesic dome Buckminster Fuller, and the U. S. economist, Kenneth Galbraith. I am often asked how it is that – nearing ninety – I seem to remain psychologically as active as ever. The reason basically is divine grace. In addition, I continue to walk half an hour every day, read a variety of books mainly the glorious Upanishads, play bridge with my computer, invariably do the Asian Age scrabble, and of course pursue my puja, pranayama and bhakti for two hours a day. Simply being a passive viewer of television may in fact have a negative impact, specially if we watch movies or serials full of violence and hatred. The internet can also be a mixed blessing and we must use it responsibly.

Finally, there is **Spiritual age**. Here we enter an ageless realm, because the spiritual quest cannot be put into a time strait jacket. The important thing is for us to realize that life is not merely a meaningless journey from the womb to the tomb, but a unique opportunity for spiritual growth. I cannot here go into this aspect in any detail, except to say that all religions speak of an inner light which represents our spiritual goal. The Bible calls it "the Light that lighteth every man that cometh into the world", Sufis call it the Noor-e-Ruhani, Sikhs call it Ek Onkar, the Vedanta calls it the Efflulgent Light of Lights. Whatever path we may be following into our old age, it is very important that elderly people do have a spiritual awareness which will be a great support and solace to them in the ageing process.

Having delineated these five dimensions of age, I must finally address the question of Death which ultimately will come to us all. The Geeta simply says "that which is born must die and that which dies must be re-born. Therefore, for what is inevitable, we should not grieve". Of course, this is easier said than done but, if possible, we should approach death with courage and dignity. This will depend to a considerable extent on how modern medicine can keep us comfortable. Geriatrics is now a specialized branch of medicine dealing exclusively with the problems of old age, and both pharmacological and handicapped-friendly products are growing rapidly. Buildings now are legally required to have special facilities for the handicapped. There is also the delicate question of giving terminally ill people the **Right to Die**. In fact, this is one of the last human rights that humanity has not yet agreed, and is the subject of an animated international controversy.

To conclude, therefore, Ageing involves coping with life and coping with death. It is our unique privilege as human beings to be aware of these challenges and to mobilize our physiological, emotional, intellectual and spiritual resources to treat ageing as a unique learning experience which helps us on our eternal spiritual quest. Let me end with a Vedic prayer for a long & vigorous life that has come down to us through the long and tortuous corridors of time for thousands of years:

"For a hundred autumns, may we see
For a hundred autumns, may we live
For a hundred autumns, may we know
For a hundred autumns, may we rise
For a hundred autumns, may we be
For a hundred autumns, may be become
Aye, and even more than a hundred autumns"

– Atharva Veda XIX, 67

2
As I Age
Sunderlal Bahuguna

मेरा जन्म रिसायत के दस परिवारों के गॉव मरोड़ा में हुआ था। यह गॉव राजा के दीवान खानदान के डोभालों का था। मेरे नाना श्री अभय डोभाल के पॉच पुत्र और दो बेटियॉ थी, जिनमें एक मेरी मॉ थी। नाना ने पिताजी के साथ शर्त रखी थी कि बेटी की शादी तुम्हारे साथ तब ही होगी जब तुम इसी गॉव में रहने को तैयार हो। मैं अपनी बेटी को अपनी जायदाद में भागीदार बनाऊंगा। उन्होंने अपनी जमीन का काफी भाग मेरी मॉ को दे दिया। हमारा पैतृक गॉव गोदी में था, वहॉ भी हमारी पर्याप्त जमीन और अच्छा मकान था, लेकिन मेरी बड़ी मॉ की सन्तान न होने से पिताजी को नाना की शर्त मंजूर कर मरोड़ा में ही बसना पड़ा। वहीं से सिल्यारा की जमीन का काम करवाते थे।

पिताजी वन विभाग में वन अधिकारी थे और मैं उनके बुढ़ापे की (59 वें)सबसे छोटी संतान था। लोग जब मुझे रेंजर साहब का बेटा कहकर पुकारते थे तो मुझे गर्व होता लेकिन जब बुढ्या जी का बेटा कहते मैं गुस्सा होता। पिताजी हर माह जब 6 किमी0 दूर घोड़े पर बैठकर पेंशन लेने जाते मुझे भी अपने साथ घोड़े पर बैठाकर टिहरी ले जाते। घोड़ा पुल पार नहीं ले जाते थे। एक दुकान के सामने बॉध देते और मुझे चना गुड़ दे जाते ताकि मैं परेशान न हो जाऊं।
घर में सबसे छोटा होने के नाते मुझे सबका प्यार दुलार मिलता था। मुझसे बड़े दो भाई और दो बहिनें थी। लेकिन जब मैं आठ साल का था पिताजी हमें छोड़कर चले गये और मॉ भी सत्रह वर्ष का छोड़कर चली गई, पर मुझे बड़े भाई–बहिनों का प्यार–दुलार मिलता रहा।
राजशाही में शिक्षा व्यवस्था नही के बराबर थी। राजा नहीं चाहते थे कि लोग शिक्षित होकर अपने अधिकारों की मांग करें, मेरी प्राईमरी तक की शिक्षा गॉव से तीन किमी0 दूर गेरण स्कूल में हुई, चौथी कक्षा की पढ़ाई के लिए अपनी दीदी के पास उत्तरकाशी चला गया। वहॉ मेरे जीजा जी (बहनोई) श्री महेशानन्द उनियाल शास्त्री जी संस्कृत के शिक्षक थे।

प्राईमरी के बाद मैं टिहरी कॉलेज में भर्ती हुआ। हाईस्कूल की परीक्षा देने दो दिन पैदल चलकर देहरादून आया। उसके बाद टिहरी इंटर तक हो गया और मैंने अपनी इंटर तक की पढ़ाई प्रताप इंटर कॉलेज से और स्नातक की शिक्षा लाहौर सनातन धर्म कॉलेज में हुई।
जब मैं 16 वर्ष का था, मेरी मुलाकात श्री देव सुमन जी से हुई। उनकी वेश–भूषा सामान्य लोगों और दरबारियों से भिन्न थी। उन दिनों सड़क पर दो ही प्रकार के लोग दिखाई देते थे, एक अचकन और चूड़ीदार पजामा पहने हुए अधिकारी और दूसरे लंगोटी पहने हुए गरीब लोग। इनसे भिन्न पहचान वाले इस युवक श्री देव सुमन ने हमको आकर्षित किया । वे खादी की सफेद टोपी , लंबा कुर्ता, धोती और चप्पल पहने हुए थे। बाजार में बरगद के पेड़ के नीचे के चबूतरे में बैठ कर दिन भर चरखा कातते थे। एक दिन मैंने जिज्ञासावश उनसे पूछा आप इस चरखे से साल भर भी कातते रहेंगे तो भी आपका इतना लंबा कुर्ता नहीं बन पायेगा। उन्होंने उत्तर दिया– मेरा कुर्ता बने न बने गॉधी जी कहते हैं कि यदि सब चरखा कातने लगें तो अंग्रेज भारत छोड़कर चले जायेंगे और हमारे देश की गरीबी मिट जायेगी । खादी के वस्त्रों से लोगों को रोजगार मिलेगा। मैंने पूछा गॉधी जी और क्या कहते हैं ? उन्होंने कहा तुम और जानना चाहते हो तो मेरे पास ये किताबें हैं

इन्हें खरीदकर पढ़ो। उन्होंने अपने झोले से दो छोटी किताबें निकाली । महात्मा गॉधी की लिखी **"हिन्द स्वराज्य"** और दूसरी प्रिंस क्रोपोटकिन की **"नवयुवकों से दो बातें"**

मेरी मॉ मुझे सप्ताह के छः दिनों के लिए 6 आने देती थी। रोज दो पैंसे का पाव भर दूध और दो पैसे की जलेबी खाने के लिए मैंने एक हफ्ते की दूध और जलेबी कुर्बान कर कर ये दोनों किताबें खरीद ली। इन किताबों ने मेरे जीवन की दिशा बदल दी। मैं राजा की नौकरी के बजाय देश को आजाद करने और दुनिया को बदलने के आन्दोलन में कूद पड़ा। मेरी खादी की सफेद टोपी और सुमन जी से संपर्क से मॉ और मामा चिन्तित रहने लगे। मॉ ने कहा तुम्हारे पिता ने दरबार का नमक खाया है इसका ध्यान रखो। बड़े मामा ने कहा यह कंस भांजा पैदा हो गया है। लेकिन हमारे सामने गॉधी की चुनौती थी, तुम गुलाम पैदा हुये हो आजाद होकर मरना। मैं बगावती हो गया । दसवीं की परीक्षा देकर सुमन जी के साथ गर्मी की छुट्टियों में मसूरी चला गया, जहॉ सुमन जी गरीब मजदूरों के लिए रात्रिशाला चलाते थे, इसी बीच मॉ चली गई। मैं प्रताप इंटर कॉलेज में पढ़ने लगा। श्री देव सुमन को राजद्रोही जेल में डाल दिया गया। कारागार में उन पर कोड़े बरसाये जाते। जेल के भीतर ही न्यायाधीश के सामने दिया गया उनका वक्तव्य और उन पर होने वाले अमानवीय व्यवहार की खबरें दिल्ली अखबारों में छपी। उस जुर्म में मुझे पकड़ा गया पर प्रधानाध्यापक के इस बयान से कि लड़का है तो गॉधी बाबा का अनुयायी परन्तु चरित्रवान व प्रतिभाशाली है, परीक्षा देने की अनुमति दी जाय। परीक्षा स्थल तक पुलिस की निगरानी में रह कर परीक्षा दी और परीक्षा सभा के बाद नरेन्द्रनगर हवालात में बंद कर दिया गया, क्योंकि टिहरी जेल में सुमन जी बन्द थे। हवालात से पॉच माह बाद डॉक्टर की रिपोर्ट के आधार छूट सारे शरीर में फोड़े हो गए थे। इस बीच सुमन जी 84 दिन के उपवास के बाद शहीद हो गए थे। राजशाही ने घबराकर मुझे डॉक्टर के आदेश पर गुम कर दिया और मैं कुछ ठीक होने पर अपने बड़े भाई गोपाल राम जी के साथ लाहौर पढ़ने चला गया। वहॉ भी राजा की पुलिस पीछा करती रही। एक साल पंजाब के लालयपुर जिले में सिख बनकर जमींदार के बेटों को पढ़ाता रहा। फिर अपनी परीक्षा देकर टिहरी लौटा और राजशाही को समाप्त करने के आन्दोलन में सक्रिय हो गया। सन 1948 में अपने दो हौनहार नौजवानों की शहादत के बाद जनता उमड़ पड़ी। टिहरी राज्य की सत्ता को जनता ने अपने हाथों में ले लिया। सन 1949 को जब मैंने गॉधी जी से मिला। अपने टिहरी की अहिंसक लड़ाई की कहानी गॉधी जी को सुनाई, उन्होंने कहा– शाबाश तुम हिमालय जितनी उंचाई पर रहते हो उतना बड़ा काम किया। मेरी अहिंसा को धरती पर ले आये। उनका यह वाक्य हमारा **पाचेय** बन गया।

हमने राजनीतिक आजादी प्राप्त कर ली लेकिन सामाजिक समानता , अस्पृश्यता का रोग, आर्थिक असमानता , शराब से बरबादी आदि समस्याओं से जूझने के लिए लोक शक्ति जगाने का वृहद काम सामने था। नगर के सफाई कर्मियों की बस्ती में रात को नशे में लड़ाई झगड़े होते थे, गन्दगी निरक्षरता थी। हमने शुरूआत रात्रि में बस्ती में प्रार्थना एवं शिक्षण कार्य से की। उनमें बदलाव होने लगा शिक्षा के प्रति उनमें जागरूकता पैदा हुई।

गांधी जी ने कहा था राजनैतिक स्वतंत्रता हासिल करने के बाद जागरूक लोगों को लोक शक्ति जगाने व गॉवों को आत्मनिर्भर बनाने, गॉव की समस्याओं को गॉव में ही हल करने में अपनी शक्ति लगानी चाहिए। सत्ता को विकेन्द्रीत कर, गॉवों को पंचायतों को मजबूत कर केन्द्रित सत्ता पर निर्भरता कम से कम होनी चाहिए। हमारा सौभाग्य था कि गांधी जी की दो अंग्रेज अनुयायी **"मीराबाई"** एवं **"सरला बहन"** का मार्गदर्शन हमें मिला। हमारी रिसायत में उच्च शिक्षा की व्यवस्था नहीं थी, लड़कियों के लिए तो शिक्षा के दरवाजे बन्द थे । केवल एक आठवीं का स्कूल नगर में था। विमला नौटियाल के भाई ने जो खुद स्वतंत्रता सेनानी थे, ने विमला को सरला बहन के पास शिक्षण के लिए भेजा, जहॉ उनके सानिध्य में उन्हें शिक्षा के साथ सामाजिक समस्याओं के लिए लोक शक्ति जगाकर समस्याओं के समाधन की प्रेरणा मिली, और उन्होंने शादी के प्रस्ताव पर राजनीति का रास्ता छोड़कर गॉवों को केन्द्र बनाकर कार्य करने की शर्त रखी। हम दोनों ने दूरस्थ क्षेत्र सिल्यारा को अपना कार्य क्षेत्र बनाकर कार्य प्रारंभ किया। गॉधी ने कहा था मेरा जीवन ही मेरा संदेश है। हम जिन मूल्यों को समाज में कायम करना चाहते हैं स्वयं पहले अपने जीवन में उतारें। गांधी जी ऐसा भारत बनाना चाहते थे जिसमें सत्ता, सम्पत्ति व शस्त्र के स्थान पर सेवा, त्याग व शांति प्रेम की प्रतिष्ठा हो। भारी भरकम केन्द्रित सरकार के बजाय गॉव में आपसी प्रेम सदभावपूर्ण स्वावलम्बी समाज हो।

हम लोगों ने तय किया कि हम अपनी आवश्यकताएँ कम से कम रखेंगे, श्रमनिष्ठ जीवन और गलत मान्यताओं को बदलने को लोगों को प्रेरित करें। शादी में समाज में दहेज दावत दिखावे पर अंकुश लगे। हमने अपनी शादी में केवल अड़तालीस रूपये खर्च किये। शास्त्रीय विधि के अलावा वृक्षारोपण, यज्ञ, सफाई, भोजन, मिठाई के स्थान पर गुड़ देकर ये नई परंपरा लोगों के बीच कायम की और यह तय किया कि हम उसी शादी में शामिल होंगे जहॉ सादगी से दहेज दावत का अनावश्यक आडम्बर नहीं होगा और जीवनभर इस नियम पर कायम रहें । सौभाग्य से हम दोनों के परिवार ने हमें भरपूर सहयोग व प्यार दिया, तभी हम अपने जीवन में समाज में जागरूकता पैदा करने का कुछ–कुछ कार्य कर पाये। हमने अपने जीवन यापन के लिए बाहरी सहायता न लेकर खुद श्रमनिष्ठ जीवन जीने का तय किया। मुझे अखबारों में समाचार भेजने से थोड़ी आय होती थी अपने लिए दूध सब्जी, फल हम खुद पैदा कर लेते थे। अनाज की पूर्ति गॉव के परिवार फसल पर हमें धन, गेहूँ इकट्ठा कर देते थे। वे हमारे परिवारें से परिचित थे। उन्हें पता था ये संपन्न परिवार से पढ़ लिखकर अच्छी नौकरी न कर हमारे बीच आये है।

हम शाम की प्रार्थना गॉव में सामूहिक रूप से बैठकर करते। प्रार्थना के साथ सामूहिक सूत कताई का कार्य भी चलता। मैं सामूहिक रूप से समस्याओं पर चर्चा कर उनके समाधान पर चर्चा करता किशारों को पढ़ाता। विमला आश्रम में जा कर लड़कियों को पढ़ाती। उनमें छुआछूत , स्त्री शक्ति जागरण आदि पर चर्चा करती। इससे उनमें आत्मविश्वास बढ़ता। लड़कियॉ शाम के भोजन के लिए अपने साथ खाना लेकर आती तो सब मिलकर खाते, छुआछूत का भेद सहज रूप से उनके मन से निकलता जाता। माताएं शुरू में लडकियों को पढाई को कहती, इन्हें घास ही तो काटनी है, पहले भाई बहिनों की देखभाल फिर गाय भैंस के लिए चारा लाने में मॉ का हाथ बंटाना। इसलिए हमने रात्रिशाला से शुरूआत की। हम भी उन्हीं की तरह अपने आश्रम में खेती, गोपालन व साथ में शिक्षण कार्य भी करते। आश्रम को हमने गॉव के लिए एक प्रयोगशाला व अपने लिए साधन स्थल माना था। हम उन्हें अन्य के साथ स्वस्थ जीवन के लिए सब्जी, फल, भाजी, संतुलित आहार की आवश्यकता समझाते। फसल पर सब्जी के बीच लाकर उन्हें देते।

इस प्रकार किसी गृहस्थी के कार्यों के साथ सामाजिक समस्याओं पर भी चर्चा में भागीदारी करने को बहिनों को प्रेरित करते। धीरे–धीरे तीन बहिनों ने अपनी समस्याएँ उजागर करनी शुरू की। हम शराब से दुखी हे, परिवार में कलह, समाज में माहौल खराब हो जाता है। आर्थिक बर्बादी की जड़ तो है ही।

हमने उन्हें प्रेरित किया , हम सबने मिलकर गांव में बनने वाली शराब के अड्डों पर जाकर उन्हें समाप्त करने के कार्य में जब उन्हें सफलता मिली फिर उन्होंने सरकार की दुकानों पर धरना देकर उन्हें बंद करने का मोर्चा संभाला। वे अपने डेढ़ साल, तीन साल, छः साल के बच्चों को लेकर जेलों में गई । शराब को महिला शक्ति के दबाव पर सरकार को उत्तराखंड में सब दुकानें बंद करनी पड़ी।

बहिनों को अपनी सामूहिक शक्ति का एहसास हुआ। उन्हें भरोसा हुआ कि वे समाज और सरकार के गलत निर्णयों को सामूहिक शक्ति द्वारा बदलने में भागीदारी निभा सकती है।

फिर तो उन्होंने जंगलों के द्वारा होने वाले विनाश को रोकने के लिए पेड़ों को कटने से बचाने का मोर्चा संभाला, जिसके लिए उन्हें महीने भर भी जंगलों में डेरे डालने पड़े। बडियारगढ के मालगडडी के जंगल में हमारे आश्रम के पास के क्षेत्र से वहॉ की बहिनों को मदद करने छः बहिनें पूरे महीने भर कटने वाले वन में डेरा डालकर कटाई बंद होने के आदेश पर ही लौटी।

पेडों की कटाई बंद कराने में उत्तराखंड की बहिनों को आठ वर्ष लगे। लेकिन पर्यावरण संरक्षण की इस अहिंसक प्रतिकार ने बहिनों में आत्मविश्वास जगाया। दुनिया को पेड़ों के बारे में नई दृष्टि दी।

क्या है जंगल के उपकार
मिट्टी पानी और बयार,
मिट्टी पानी और बयार
जिंदा रहने के आधार।

पेड़ों की कटाई पर प्रतिबंध लगने से बौंखलाए वन विभाग ने लोगों को सबक सिखाने की नीयत से लोगों को रियायती दर पर हक हकूक की लकड़ी देना बंद कर दिया। सिल्यारा गॉव की अनपढ़ डॉक्टर बच्चों की जड़ी बूटियों से उपचार में माहिर क्रांतिकारी महिला जुपली देवी अपने महिला समूह के साथ चीड़ की लकड़ी की मसाल लेकर 12 बजे दोपहर रयाला चौकी रेंज ऑफिसर के कार्यालय पहुँची। हमारे लिए स्वराज्य नहीं अंधेरे का राज हो गया है। वनों को पालने वाली जनता को पीडियों से मिलने वाले हक हकूक भी बंद हो गये हैं। गरीब की झोपड़ी के लिए लकड़ी नहीं। सूखी गिरी लकड़ी वन निगम बनाकर टुकड़ा टुकड़ा बाहर ले जाया जाता है। हमें घास लकड़ी के लिए मीलों की दूरी तय करनी पड़ती है।
उन्होंने गाना शुरू कर दिया।

खड़ा उठा भाई बहणों, सब कट्ठा होला
सरकारी नीति से जंगल बचोला,
सरकार मालदार पैंसा कमौंदा
पहाड़ी छोटा भैर भांडा मठौंदा,
भाई बहिनों जाग जाओं ,

सरकार व ठेकेदार जंगलों से पैंसे कमाकर मालदार हो रहे हैं। हमारे बच्चे रोजगार की तलाश में बाहर शहरों में बर्तन मांजने को मजबूर है।

घास, लाखड़ु मादु पांणी
यूं का बिना योजना कांणी

यानि जिन योजनाओं में घास, लकड़ी, मिट्टी पानी को प्राथमिकता नहीं, हमारे लिए वह योजना अंधी अनुपयोगी है। महिलाओं की बातें सुनकर रेंज ऑफिस को पसीना छूट गया। दो घंटे तक वह अपनी कुर्सी पर न बैठ सका, खड़ा–खड़ा आश्वासन देता रहा। मेरे अधिकार में आने वाली मॉगों को अवश्य पूरा करूंगा। महिलाओं ने मॉग पत्र रखा–

बिन्दु 1–वनों की नीति तय करने में पहाड़ की जनता की भागीदारी हो।
बिन्दु 2–सूखी गिरी पड़ी लकड़ी पहले आम आदमी के उपयोग के लिए हो।
बिन्दु 3–वनों के वृक्षारोपण में महिलाओं की भागीदारी हो, ताकि हमें पता हो कि किस प्रजाति के पेड़ लगाये जा रहे हैं।
बिन्दु 4–महिलाओं का जीवन वनों से जुड़ा है। उनकी कष्ट मुक्ति वाले पौष्टिक चारे के पेड़ तथा पानी के स्त्रोत बढ़ाने को प्राथमिकता दी जाय ताकि महिलाओं को घास लकड़ी के लिए मीलों दूर न जाना पड़े। हमारा पूरा समय इसमें जाता है कि बच्चों के व अपने बौद्विक विकास के लिए समय नहीं मिल पाता है।

इस मुहिम के परिणामस्वरूप वनों की नर्सरी तैयार करके वृक्षारोपण में महिलाओं की नियुक्ति हुई। आस–पास वातावरण में जागरूकता के अलावा हम लोग पैदल यात्राओं के द्वारा पहाड़ के दूरस्थ क्षेत्रों तक महिला शक्ति जागरण, व्यसन मुक्ति एवं पर्यावरण संरक्षण एवं समाज की समस्याओं को सुलझाने में लोक शक्ति जगाने की दृष्टि से कार्य करते रहे।

इनमें महिलाओं की भी बराबर भागीदारी रही। सरला बहन की हीरक जयंती पर बहिनों ने पूरे उत्तराखंड की यात्रा निकाली थी और पेड़ों के कटान पर प्रतिबंध लगाने पर मैंने कश्मीर से कोहिमा 4,870(चार हजार आठ सौ सत्तर) किमी0 की पैदल यात्रा द्वारा लोक शक्ति जागरण हेतु की। अस्पृश्यता निवारण के लिए हम लोगों ने सभी को साथ लेकर मन्दिर प्रवेश के कार्य द्वारा जागृति के प्रयास किये। आज जीवन के चौथे पड़ाव पर पहुँच गया। हम शारीरिक कमजोरी के बावजूद मन से प्रसन्न व संतुष्ट है। हमें संतोष है कि हमने अपने जीवन के प्रत्येक क्षण का सदुपयोग किया। समाज के आम आदमी की तरह अपना स्वावलंबी जीवन जी कर शोषण व शासनमुक्त समाज बनाने के लिए लोक शक्ति, आत्मशक्ति जगाने का प्रयास किया।

हमने समाज में जिन मूल्यों को अपनाने को कहा उसके अनुरूप जीवन बिताया। हमारे तीनों बच्चों का शिक्षण गॉव के बच्चों की तरह उन्हीं के साथ हुआ। उच्च शिक्षा भी टिहरी, पौड़ी व उत्तरकाशी के पहाड़ी क्षेत्रों में हुई।

अब हम अपने हमउम्र साथियों, महानुभावों से निवेदन करते हैं कि उम्र के इस पड़ाव पर पहुँचकर शारीरिक कमजोरियों को जीवन की एक प्रकिया मानकर प्राणायाम, आसन एवं सारे सुपाच्य भोजन द्वारा बीमारियों से शरीर को बचाने का प्रयास करें। अपना समय आध्यत्मिक साहित्य पढ़ने, दूरदर्शन पर अच्छे कार्यक्रम देखने व एक दूसरे के साथ प्रेमपूर्वक व्यवहार में बिताएँ। नित्य कुछ समय पैदल घूमें।

मेरे पास आज भी देश दुनिया से लोग आते हैं। उन्हें मार्गदर्शन देने में मुझे आनन्द महसूस होता है। मैं उनसे कहता हूँ कि हमारे राष्ट्रीय गान में जैसे सुजलांम, सुफलाम, मलयजशीतलाम की प्रार्थना की गई है हम अपनी प्रकृति को हरे भरे प्रदूषण मुक्त बनाने का प्रयास करें।

हम उस संस्कृति के वाहक है जहॉ ऋषियों ने "बसुदैव कुटुम्बकम" का मंत्र हमें दिया है। आज के युग के ऋषि विनोबा ने तो अभिवादन में ही जय जगत का मंत्र देकर हमें जागरूक किया है।

यानि हम अपने को, मैं तक सीमित नहीं पूरे विश्व का अंग मानकर उस प्रभु का धन्यवाद करें जिसने हमें ऐसी संस्कृति संपन्न भारत भूमि में जन्म दिया।

राज्य मॉगू नहीं, स्वर्ग मॉगू नहीं
मुक्ति की नींद में क्या मजा है
दीन के दुख भव, क्षय मिटाया करें
दीन बन्धु यही वर मुझे दो

अपने जीवन के संघर्षों में भी इस भावना से हमें बल मिलता रहा है। अपने भारत की गौरवपूर्ण संस्कृति की विरासत को हम कुछ हद तक अपने जीवन में जी पाएँ इसका हमें परम संतोष है। इंसान में कुछ कमियॉ और अच्छाईयॉ होती हैं। हम दोनों ने अपने जीवन में एक दूसरे की कमियों पर कभी ध्यान न देकर अच्छाईयों को आगे बढ़ने का मौका दिया। इससे हमारे जीवन में कभी कटुता और तनाव का वातावरण नहीं रहा, आज भी एक–दूसरे की रूचि का पूरा ध्यान रख कर अपनी दिनचर्या निभाते हैं तो दोनों प्रसन्न व आनन्द में रहते हैं। रात को अच्छी नींद आती है।*

---

* Sunderlal Bahuguna passed away on 21st May 2021 at the age of 94. This Hindi article was one of the last pieces hand-written by him.

English Translation

I was born in the village of Marorain Garhwal in present day Uttarakhand. My maternal grandfather Shri Abhay Ram Dobhal had five sons and two daughters. He had abundant land. My father was from Sirar Godi. He was a forest range officer. His first wife had no children. When a proposal came from him to my maternal grandfather the latter put a condition that his daughter would get married to him only if my father would live in his village. He promised to give adequate land to his daughter. My father accepted the conditions and made Marora his home. We were three brothers and two sisters. I was the youngest and enjoyed the love of my parents and all my older siblings. We lost our father when I was 8 years old. Educational facilities were scarce during the rule of the Tehri king. I did my primary schooling in a village 3 km away. I then moved to Uttarkashi to stay with my older sister to study up to Class 9. Her husband was my teacher.

When I was 13, I met Sri Dev Suman. He was dressed differently from others in a white kurta and dhoti made of khadi. He carried a box with him always and I was curious to know the contents of the box. He opened the box, took out a charkha and started spinning. I told him that even if he spun for a whole year, he would not be able to spin enough for his long kurta. He said, "The issue is not how long it will take to spin enough cloth for my kurta. I spin because Gandhi has told us that we will only get freedom from the British if every Indian spins. Khadi gives work to people. Work will remove poverty."

I asked, "What else did Gandhi say?"

He advised me to buy and read the books he had written.

My mother used to give me some pocket money for milk and jalebis. I spent one week's money on two books. The first was Gandhi's *Hind Swara*. The second was Prince Kropotkin's *My Appeal to Youth*.

These two books changed the direction of my life. Instead of trying to look for a job in the King's government, I jumped into the freedom movement for the Independence of the country and transformation of the world, to remove injustice. I started to wear the white cap of our freedom fighters. Seeing my closeness to Sri Dev Suman, my mother and maternal uncle started to get anxious. My mother said, "Remember, your father worked for the King".

But I had heard Gandhi's call "You were born in slavery, you must die in freedom". I became a rebel.

When I was 17, my mother passed on.

I continued my association with Suman. While I was studying in inter college, Suman was arrested for rebelling against the king. His declaration, when the sentence passed against him was jail, made it to the Delhi papers. I was arrested in connection with spreading the news of Suman's arrest. I took my examination under police supervision. After my examination I was taken to Narendranagar jail. Suman was in Tehri jail. They gave me three rotis per day. During the five months of being in prison, I became very sick. My body was covered with boils. I was taken to the hospital, and the doctor advised complete rest. He also advised that I should be allowed to become better before taking me back to the jail. The authorities let me go, apprehensive that I might die in prison. I escaped to Lahore where I started studying for my Bachelors' Degree. The King's police came looking for me in Lahore. I went into hiding in Lyallpur as "Sardar Man Singh"wearing a turban. To earn a living, I taught the children of a local Zamindar. After completing my degree, I returned to Tehri. In 1948, our region gained independence from the rule of the King. Two youths lost their lives in fighting for freedom.

There was anger among the public. Through non-violence the people took over the governance of Tehri. On 29th Jan I met Gandhiji to get his blessings. He said: "You have brought my dream of non-violent resistance to the mountains". His blessings became my strength. We had gained political freedom, but social injustices continued. We had the big challenge of empowering women, removing caste discrimination, and addressing the issue of alcoholism. We started a major campaign for social awareness.

Gandhi had said that, after political independence, people with a social conscience should work to make the villages self-reliant (AtmaNirbhar). We were blessed to get the guidance of two of Gandhi's followers – Mira Behn and Sarala Behn. Bimla my future wife had studied with Sarla Behn in Laxmi Ashram where, besides education, she learnt how to work with women to empower them and build people's movements. I worked to edit Mira Behn's newsletter *Bapu Raj* when she started her centre in Gewli village in Bhilangana. Her simplicity and high ideas influenced me greatly. After Independence, I became the secretary of the District Congress Committee and Harijan Sewa Sangh. I started campaigns for temple entry for Harijans. When I proposed marriage to Bimla, she put a condition that she would agree to marry me if I left the path of politics and made service to the villages the focus of my work.

Gandhi said, "My life is my message". In other words, make the values you want to see in society the values by which you live your life. Gandhi wanted to create an India based not on power and property but on service, love, peace, simplicity, and restraint. He wanted to create an India free of exploitation.

Bimla and I got married with Rs 30. We did not allow waste or dowry., We decided to minimise our needs and do physical work. Our wedding ceremony included planting trees and cleaning our environment. We distributed gur instead of sweets and started a new tradition of celebration with simplicity. We decided to attend only weddings that had no dowry, no wasteful expenditure. Our three children got married without dowry in the Shivanand Ashram in Rishikesh.

Our work was based on self-reliance and our own efforts, not on external support. I earned some money as a journalist writing for newspapers. We grew our own vegetables, raised our cows, produced our milk. The village community shared food grains with us in exchange for our labour. Every evening we held a collective prayer meeting in the village. We would spin collectively and discuss social problems. During the day I would teach village boys. In the evening Bimla taught the girls after they finished working in the fields with their mothers. While teaching them Bimla would also discuss social ills and unjust traditions. Their confidence in themselves started to grow. They brought their evening meal with them and shared the meal. Through eating together, all caste discrimination started to disappear.

The Silyara Ashram we started was an experiment of social justice for the village community. For us it was our site and mode of meditation. We lived and farmed like the villagers while carrying out our community education work. We distributed vegetable seeds, and encouraged women to participate in social issues. Slowly they became active in articulating their problems. They said, "Alcohol has destroyed our homes and society". We inspired them to join hands and address the problem collectively. First, they shut down a liquor unit that was being set up in the village. Then they started to protest at government liquor shops. With their little children they went to jail. Shutting down liquor shops made them aware of their power. They realized that we can change the wrong policies of government and wrong policies of society with our collective power.

Then the women turned their attention to stop the commercialization of forestry and prevent the ecological destruction it was causing. The Chipko movement led by women gave a new perspective on trees and forests to the world.

Their collective message was:
What are the gifts of the forest?
Soil, water and pure air.
Soil, water and air are the basis of life
"The axes can be sharpened, but we will hug the trees
We will face sticks and bullets
To protect our trees.

It took eight years of camping in forests to prevent logging of green trees. By 1981, we achieved a ban on logging.

The Silyara Ashram became a centre of our activism on temple-entry, Chipko, and women's equality. We undertook padyatras for ecological and social awareness. After we got a logging ban, I undertook a Himalayan padyatra from Kashmir to Kohima to raise environmental awareness. I walked 4,877 kms across the Himalayas with young activists.

I am now in the fourth stage of my life. While my body is feeble, my mind is active, my heart is full of joy and satisfaction. We have the satisfaction that we have used every moment of our lives for the larger social good, and made the social values of justice and equality the basis of our lives and our struggles. Our children studied with the village children.

The inspiration that has given us strength throughout our lives is this:

I don't seek the throne, I don't seek heaven,
The sleep of freedom brings such solace,
Removing the pain of the downtrodden.
Deenbandhu, give me this blessing".

To our fellow travellers who have reached the fourth stage of life like us, accept the frailty of the body as part of life. Simple food, pranayama, and a little walking gives you strength.

Read spiritual texts, watch good programmes on Doordarshan, and relate to those around you with love.

People from across the world still come to visit me. I enjoy sharing my life's experience with them. Like the words of our national song, "Sujalam, Sufalam, Maliyaj Sithalam", we should make every effort to protect nature and create a pollution-free environment. A simple life according to the values of Indian Ecological Civilisation can show the way.

We all have weaknesses. Bimla and I have not paid attention to each other's weaknesses. We have encouraged the goodness in each other to grow and flourish. That is why there has never been tension and negativity in our relationship. Even today we take care of each other and spend our days together.

We live in joy and peace, we sleep well.

May God continue to bless us.

3
Let Go
Dr. V. Mohini Giri

Many of my well wishers often ask me, "How old are you?" I tell them:

How can I answer
This stupid question?
When I play with a little child
I am one year old.
When I watch cartoons
I'm three.
When I dance to the tune of music, I am sweet sixteen.
Yes, when I try to heal
Someone's wound,
I'm sure I've crossed six decades of my life span.
And when I chat with sparrows or bulbuls,
Or run after my dog and his ball
I become their age.

What is there in age?
Isn't it a number only?
Like the light of the sun
And the flowing river waters
I am ageless.
I keep changing with time and experience.
Days are marching towards night.
No doubt,

Whenever it extends its hand
I shall hold it.
Till then it's not my age that matters.
How fully have I lived thus far?
That is the consideration.

– Mario de Andrade

It was in 1971 that I realized that only way to be happy is to **Let go**. My mother, who was a pillar of strength to me, left the world at the age of fifty-four. That incident told me that life is not about worrying, life is not about stress, but life is to be lived, loved, and let go. I also realised that the letting go involves giving up old habits, passions, to move forward or evolve to the next step and above all to compromise. From childhood I was brought up with a strong set of values, especially where elders were concerned. Respect them. Speak the truth whatever the consequences are. Help everyone and anyone if it is in one's capacity without any selfish motives. My mother would say, "*Rishtey jodo mat todo*" (make, don't break relationships)

My father died long ago in 1951 leaving behind my thirty-four year old mother with seven children. My mother ensured that we kept in touch with the elders of our paternal side of the family. She often ticked me off even when I was an adult if I failed to call my paternal uncles or aunts on a regular basis. What taught me how important it is to show love and affection to the elderly? Even today at the age of 83, I continue to enjoy a beautiful relationship with my siblings, my cousins and my in-laws and the world family at large. That made me realize if you give a little love to your elders, you get back 100 times and more from them. I was taught to invest in love, accumulate affection and get manifold dividends. My mother's guidance in my school and college made me a very confident person. My father-in-law President V. V. Giri and my mother-in-law Smt. Saraswati Giri fought for India's freedom. They were often jailed, penniless, yet they were living examples of growing old.

I had my friends in the college with the same mindset and upbringing. So, our love and respect for our senior teachers, our college hostel staff, Gulab Singh our waterman, and our cooks was the same, with no difference. Neither did we see any difference of caste, creed, religion, or economic status. It was an idyllic world, with no violence of action or words to mar it. Today I also know how important it is for friends to meet often and sit down and chat with each other. Ageing with strangers is not the same as ageing with friends. Sometime ago when I was 50 years old and my children had grown up, I started meeting my college friends more often. We were very fortunate in getting values of positive thinking right from the beginning. Each student had an advisor who would counsel us and guide us on the values of love, care, and share. These values, from Principal to staff and the 4th class staff were the pillar of strength for us. For example, when we all met in the dining room, we had to maintain strict discipline. Ten girls sat on a table, and we would elect a Head for each table. The Head would see that we didn't bother the kitchen staff, didn't waste food, and that no one went hungry. This bonding resulted in positive thinking and today at the age of 80 all of us enjoy meeting very often. It was that bond of friendship where everybody was equal. We alumnae of our college (Isabella Thoburn College) who are in Delhi decided that instead of whiling away our time in useless activities, we should open a school for underprivileged children, so that we justify the motto of our college: "We receive to give." Lo and behold our project started immediately and today after 20 years we look back with such great satisfaction of doing something together to improve the lives of millions of marginalized children. Today our hearts swell up in pride when we see children of our school, Social Outreach Foundation, who are occupying places in engineering, arts, sports, and music.

This may be intriguing to some; however, a bond of friendship plays a very important part for a happy old age. I can say with a great amount of certainty and satisfaction that the vast body of love among friends is very rejuvenating. Hence, being together, working together makes a special category of older people who are happy and satisfied:

What changed this world?
Why are our elderly not taken care of?
Why do our elderly feel left out?
Where did we go wrong?
Is the older generation or the younger at fault?

Ageing is a global phenomenon. Thanks to unprecedented public health advances and successes in many parts of the world, the proportion of aged 60 and over is growing faster than any other age group. The phenomenon of population ageing is pervasive, and affecting every man, woman, and child. The alteration of the age pyramid, however, poses a profound impact on a broad range of economic, political, and social conditions that requires urgent action. India is greying fast, with its elderly population next only to China, which has the largest number of elderly people in the world. The phenomenon of population ageing is growing in India. The government of India adopted the National Policy on Older Persons, in January1999. The policy defines a Senior Citizen or Elderly Person who is of age 60 years or above. As we retire from active work, people face a lot of insecurities such as - problems, isolation, fear, neglect, failing health, abuse, and economic insecurity.

Today I want to confine myself to those thousands of Vrindavan widows, some of whom are growing old graciously, leaving behind the unfortunate circumstances that they lived in. In the course of my work with them and in establishing a shelter home for them, I have had the opportunity of studying the process of ageing among those widows who have left their families and are living a nomadic existence in Vrindavan. Often when I go to meetings and make a policy for the elderly, I come across great deal of discussion on shelter, pension, healthcare facilities. However, these are not the only issues that make elderly happy, of course: providing them with finance and emotional security is a great step to well being. I have noticed younger widows and older widows grow old with great happiness and graciously when their minds are busy. Hence in a nutshell I would say providing employment or work, be it gardening, tailoring, wick-making or making disposable eco friendly plates gives them a sense of satisfaction and improves their health condition. They have a sense of self worth, of feeling wanted, which is vital for healthy ageing. The most important thing as we grow old is to keep our minds busy. We often think that retirement at the age of 60 is an indication that we should rest and take it easy. However, those who have seen and many more of them who have written in this book have grown old graciously and happily because they have kept themselves busy. Mind can play havoc when the body is becoming weak. The mind needs to be busy with family, friends, games, music, writing, with voluntary social work and, most importantly, eating a variety of food that the mind wants. I have experienced this in our Ashram in Madham Vrindavan where widows who are kept busy are the happiest ones.

I remember Tara Devi Maa growing old at our Ashram in Madham like a queen at the age of 100. She was happy, vibrant, and ready to do any task. She would instantly start dancing and singing the minute she would meet me and not only make herself happy but make everyone happy. Hence, we must cultivate a habit to embrace and include elderly in all our conversation and give them a feeling of being wanted. Tara was wanted by all of us. I have worked with widows for five decades, and I have felt that widowhood becomes a turning point in the lives of women because of disadvantages of their gender and their marital status. I have noticed senior citizens, both men and women, participating in early morning yoga together, forming their own groups and thereby giving enough space to leave their children to finish their chores in the morning. That is an important mantra, give space to each generation, because each generation has different priorities. It is also evident that the elderly are happiest when they are together and participate in all activities. They feel a sense of belonging.

My second observation has been that old age is stigmatized. When any human being -especially a widow- is stigmatized socially, they age fast. Hence, I would suggest that stigma attached to old age should be discarded. Why should ageism exist at all? We should do away with institutions, customs, language that under-values the contributions of the elderly. For example, elderly women bear the biggest burden of family care and are unpaid, unrecognized, unheard, and unsung. Added to this is the taunt that they are old and so useless. We have institutionalised the violative practice of ageism.

Now when I talk about stigma, I talk about the general stigmatisation of the old, whether they are men, women, or widows. The more one keeps aloof from daily chores and becomes dependent on society, friends, and children, the more they are shunned by these very people. The elderly need to change their attitude towards the young and be a part of the change that is taking place around them. Having said that, I would like to talk about my first visit to Vrindavan where I came across a dead body of a woman in the middle of a street in front of a temple. Onlookers kept seeing the body and walking past or watching the gleeful vultures and dogs attacking the body. I asked a passer by the reason for this. His reply was, "Amma, don't you see that she is a widow? Who will touch her? She is a bad omen." I was stunned, speechless and in tears. How can a human being be a bad omen? I soon arranged a relay party of some widows to take the body to the cremation ground. My mission since then has been to work against this socio-economic stigmatisation of widows. Abandoned widows and women grow old graciously if they are free of social stigmatization.

While working with the elderly widows I came across another very striking point. I used to see Prema Dasi always happy, satisfied with life, in spite of old age, lack of funds and illiteracy. So I sat down with her and asked her, "Prema what keeps you smiling all the time?" She looked at me seriously with her grey eyes and said, "If I tell you, you will think that I am a bad woman, and if I don't tell you that will hurt my spirit". I insisted and pleaded with her again. She came close to me and very quietly said, "You know I am very happy that my husband died". For some time, I just could not speak. Then I realized that freedom is vital for growing gracefully old. Prema had no worries. Her children were somewhere she did not know. She was free of all relationships and free of all the worries that accompany relationships. Hence, she felt a sense of freedom. In that freedom she was growing old without complaints. I am not suggesting for a single moment that one discards or breaks all relationships in old age. I am suggesting we should break the constricting ties that imprison our minds. Love, show affection, but selflessly without any expectation. I have myself noticed that ageing women are happier being single. While love is very important to be happy, freedom is also very important to be happy. The above freedom leads to some kind of detachment or surrender. Who does not love their children? We all do. But just as there is a thin line between need and greed, there is a thin line between *vatsalya* and *vyamoha*.

I found a position of detachment led to graceful living. Very often I have found if elderly ladies, or I suppose men also, avoid arguments, they will find a greater chance of being happy. As long as there is discussion on social, political or religious matters that is friendly and detached, it does not hurt the elderly. But if arguments become acrimonious, then relationships get strained. Hence, we must remember that keeping relationship with friends, neighbours and children keeps the elderly emotionally secure. If the elderly retain *vatsalya*, they will definitely age gracefully.

I would like to once again emphasise the importance of detachment: at a certain age we have to let go not only our ego, our children, our property, and our love to accumulate, in order to be happy.

The capacity of older people should be recognized and effectively used, within context. Often it might look difficult to bring opportunities for participation; but designing such intervention to facilitate the participation of older people is beneficial for the communities as well for the older people.

I am remembering the example of a 90-year old Czech grandma who turned her small village into her Art Gallery, by hand-painting flowers on its houses.

As I age, I have realized the true meaning of a poem by Mario De Andrade, "My soul has a hat":

I counted my years
And realized that I have
Less time to live by,
Than I have lived so far.
I feel like a child who won a pack of candies:
at first, he ate them with pleasure
But when he realized that there was little left,
he began to taste them intensely.
I have no time for endless meetings
where the statutes, rules, procedures &
internal regulations are discussed,
knowing that nothing will be done.
I no longer have the patience
To stand absurd people who,
despite their chronological age,
have not grown up.

My time is too short:
I want the essence,
my spirit is in a hurry.
I do not have much candy
In the package anymore.

I want to live next to humans,
very realistic people who know
How to laugh at their mistakes,
Who are not inflated by their own triumphs
& who take responsibility for their actions.
In this way, human dignity is defended
and we live in truth and honesty.
It is the essentials that make life useful.
I want to surround myself with people
who know how to touch the hearts of those
whom hard strokes of life
have learned to grow with sweet touches of the soul.
Yes, I'm in a hurry.
I'm in a hurry to live with the intensity
that only maturity can give.
I do not intend to waste any of the remaining desserts.
I am sure they will be exquisite,
much more than those eaten so far.
My goal is to reach the end satisfied
and at peace with my loved ones and my conscience.
We have two lives
& the second begins when you realize you only have one.

To conclude, I would say, to age graciously, health should be the top priority. Our independence is precious so we should not become a burden as we grow older. We should have kept enough finances for that independence. If you have finances and good health, you earn the respect of the family. Never take it for granted that your children will take care of you. As I have said earlier, we need to detach from our attachments.

To me personally, working for the marginalized has given me great satisfaction between sixty to eighty-two years of age. Single, with children far away, work and friends have kept me busy.

So, to all I say, yesterday is a cancelled cheque, tomorrow is a promissory note, today is cash. Live today fully.

4
Retrospections During the Pandemic
Tara Gandhi Bhattacharjee

I am in deep pain for millions and millions of persons across the world who have been faced with unbelievable and immeasurable suffering. I express my heartfelt appreciation and gratitude for all who are risking their lives to help and serve the needy and the society. We are together in prayer.

I want to share the following thoughts:

The pandemic of coronavirus has shattered the human soul. The cosmic law of justice has pronounced an unprecedented and unexpected fury on the human race. But this cosmic fury has awakened damaged and anguished human souls to another reality of spiritual realization of human concern.

For years now, my mind and soul have been disturbed and challenged by a certain question. I want to share this challenging thought. I have been feeling for some years now that human beings are certainly not the most important life in the creation. It is a human being's concept that the human life is the most superior. Even at the highest intellectual and spiritual level, human beings can only think and act within the limitations of the human mind. What do we know about other lives? Whether insect life, animal life, plant life or the environment, we know nothing about how plants speak to each other or how animals and insects communicate with each other. What is their philosophy? We know nothing. At least we know that we know nothing about other lives.

It is very humbling that if humankind is wiped out on this planet, the environment will not miss us at all. In fact, the environment and every other form of life will be happy without us. This pandemic has really proved that nature can live beautifully without the existence of human beings.

Even from my modest house, I am suddenly able to see so many rare flowers with lovely fragrance. I can also hear in my house the various chirpings of lovely birds which I had not heard before. It delights my heart and soul to see beautiful and rare birds in the little courtyard of my house. With the emergence of the purity of fear-free nature and environment, human beings are also perceiving the awakening of the human soul with the greatest compassion for one another, and all life. In order to bring some cheer around me and for others, I have been telling my friends on the phone, "At this stage in my life, I have finally found a companion of life. He is called Mr. Isolation."

"Mr. Isolation" has inspired me to further introspection. The entire creation is wrapped in a cosmic net. Destiny is playing with the warp and the weft of the cosmic net. While destiny is playing its game, we as human beings will have to remain with compassion and non-violence towards each other and to every life. We are all together in a spiritual awakening with the consciousness of human conscience.

Man pollutes the four elements, earth, water, fire and air. With the negativity and violence of our mind, we can also pollute space. Let us not pollute this fifth element - space. His Holiness Pope Francis once repeatedly said in a public audience, in five different languages, "The creator forgives us always, but what is created never forgives." Let us work together, and do our best, for a future where every life respects all other forms of life. Let us work towards a world where the human mind is without violence and the environment is without pollution.

5

AGEING POSITIVELY, PRODUCTIVELY AND GRACEFULLY: A MILITARY PERSPECTIVE

LT. GENERAL (RETD.) VIJAY OBEROI

Aging is a universal phenomenon that starts at birth, but the general understanding is that it is the start of the process of old age. That itself is a dilemma because no hard and fast rules exist, even for entering old age or transiting from middle age to old age. It also differs from person to person, as some age earlier and faster than others, for a variety of reasons, which we will not discuss here.

Life can be categorised in three ways. The first is obviously biological, which is based on one's date of birth. We don't have control over this. The second is determined by health condition. One can take care of health with good diet, exercise, a cheerful attitude and activity filled vocations. The third is psychological, which depends on how old one feels. Positive thinking, active life and optimistic attitude can reverse the psychological age.

According to Hindu Scriptures, life is divided into four age-based life-stages. These are Brahmcharya (student), Grihista (householder), Vanaprastha (retired) and Sannyasa (renunciation). While broadly they are applicable even today, the discussion here will necessarily be based on the present times, where the last two stages seem to have merged. In addition, the environment and lifestyles have changed and there is no common template for all.

For the purpose of this essay, I have chosen the date of retirement as laid down for government officials, which also coincides with one being categorised as a 'senior citizen' in one's own country, viz. 60 years, as the age of change.

In the military, we have Principles of War, which do not change, but one's adherence to them saves lives and brings victory. In a similar manner, we can perhaps list the following important attitudinal points for "ageing gracefully":

- accept the complexity that comes with longevity as yet another challenge.
- develop a positive attitude toward growing older.
- exercise our minds. Cerebral growth happens when we challenge our learning and stretch our thinking.
- broaden our interests. Our brains love stimulation. The result is a healthier, sharper mind.
- recognize and express gratitude. The impact that gratitude has on the quality of life is overwhelming.

Ageing is also relative, and everyone has different perceptions of ageing gracefully. While this narrative will be based on how I dealt with ageing in a positive manner, it applies to most military officers, with a few exceptions.

I had joined the National Defence Academy (NDA) Khadakvasla as a 16-year-old and when I retired at the age of 60 years, I had been 'in uniform' for over 44 years, which is the bulk of one's life! Hence, every aspect of ageing gracefully and positively has been influenced by my service in the army.

When I passed out after three years of rigorous training in NDA and another year of the same in the Indian Military Academy (IMA) Dehradun, the army had transformed me from a boy to 'an officer and a gentleman' and before I took the last step as a Gentleman Cadet, I was again reminded of the credo that all military officers follow throughout their service and even as veterans. The credo is:

"The safety honour and welfare of the country
comes first, always and every time.
The honour, welfare, and comfort of the men
you command come next.
Your own ease, comfort and safety come last,
always and every time".

– Lt Gen Field Marshal Philip Chetwode

On retirement, the second line of the credo changes to: "*The honour, welfare and comfort of the weak and needy come next.*"

In addition, on commissioning as a military officer, you are also transformed into "*An Officer and a Gentleman*", for that is what our training academies accomplish. This phrase needs to be fully understood, for there are many who do not know the nuances of this phrase. It may be noted that it is not gender specific, and women joining the military are referred to as "*Lady Officers*". When the phrase originated in England, the distinction between gentlemen and commoners was important. However, being a gentleman is no longer associated with being a man of high social position and wealth. One does not need to look any further than the media to know that "*money and power do not buy class*"! Today, being a gentleman is a matter of choice. It is a title you earn through an unwavering commitment to invest in your character. It is not about perfection, but a constantly renewed pursuit of excellence. Gentlemen are not stiff, pretentious, or focused on elevating themselves. Instead, they strive to succeed while helping those around them succeed as well. Being a gentleman means that you care about how your choices impact others. In short, it is about the 'human connection'.

Having become 'an officer and a gentleman or lady', the qualities one has imbibed and practised remain with you throughout your life. Hence, it is comparatively easy for us to transit effortlessly into the ageing process. While one is in service, the types of challenges one confronts are different than those that come one's way after we hang up our uniforms, only the setting changes and one has more time to ponder over the problem than in our younger days.

Having dealt with the preliminaries, allow me to briefly narrate salient points about my life so that what follows thereafter is seen in its correct perspective.

The first 'defining moment' in my life was the madness of the partition of our country in 1947. Our huge country was cut arbitrarily, and new nations were carved out, generating violence at an unprecedented scale. We were in the midst of that mindless violence, and had to leave home and hearth and become refugees in our own country! But we quickly stood back on our feet and in time became part of the mainstream! There are three major lessons I learnt from this horrific experience among many others. These are 'standing on your own feet'; 'the power of bonding'; and 'never give up'. These assist throughout one's life and make one stronger to cope with the vicissitudes of life.

My character was moulded by both my forward-thinking family and two schools. These were the Nazareth Academy, Gaya (Bihar), a Catholic School, run by Irish-American nuns; and Shri Ram Ashram High School, Amritsar (Punjab). They were starkly different, but they jointly infused self-confidence in me and prepared me for the challenges of life in the best possible manner. Both schools were co-educational, but where the former had its focus on European and American History and Geography; English; Shakespeare (yes, we did *The Merchant of Venice* in Class VI); the Bible and prayers in the School Chapel; the latter was traditionally Indian; focusing on dharma; Tagore; Indian values and ethics; Indian music and Art; Indian history and geography; civics (alas a forgotten subject now!); and the morning commenced with patriotic songs, bhajans or the recital of poems. I am convinced that this combination of a supportive home environment and the learning and character qualities imbibed in the schools I attended were responsible for my facing life's many challenges in my later life.

The second 'defining moment' of my life was losing my right leg on account of the severe wounds I had suffered during the war with Pakistan in 1965. The operations in various hospitals including the last one at Pune, along with getting an artificial limb, took nearly a year. During this interregnum, two major decisions shaped my later life. The first was to 'soldier-on' in my own battalion and compete with my peers in all respects. No concessions were asked for or given. The second was the culmination of a blossoming romance with the lovely and brave Daulat Surve, the daughter of the first Indian commanding officer of my battalion, which culminated in our wedding after a year! She has been the best partner I could have hoped for. She has proved to be a real 'daulat' (wealth) both in name and deed. At that juncture of my life, my 25th birthday was still over a month away; I held the rank of captain and proudly displayed the accoutrements of my regiment. I had a little over four years commissioned service and had already been blooded in battle twice, first during operations against the Portuguese in 1961 and now in the skirmish with Pakistani soldiers. The future looked uncertain, but optimism and a zest for life propelled me to "Look at the sunlight, not the shadows".

Let me now take a huge leap to 30 September 2001, over 35 years later, when I retired as Vice Chief of Army Staff of the Indian Army. I sat behind the wheel of my Toyota Corolla of 1981 vintage, flying my rectangular three-star flag for the last time, with my lady love and our two dogs besides me and headed for our newly-constructed home at Panchkula, exulting in soldiering-on in the army, which took me from a one-legged captain to the rarified heights of the second highest appointment in the Indian Army, having broken many glass ceilings on the way.

This was the start of my second career, viz. ageing positively, productively, and gracefully. I had already decided that I would not pick up a job, like many of my friends and colleagues had done, as having reached nearly at the top in the army, no job except as the head of a major organization was worth considering.

Selection of a place to settle down is an important component of ageing well. We had selected Panchkula as it met most of our requirements. These included proximity to a big military station which would enable us to continue enjoying some military facilities; having friends and relatives nearby; a comparatively new city without the woes of old established cities; well-connected and so on.

One of the first actions we took was discarding the trappings of power and ego that is part of it. The next was the setting up of a non-government organization (NGO) to assist all war disabled personnel of the three Services, to make them financially independent so that they can live with dignity and become better citizens of the country. Thus, the War Wounded Foundation was born in 2002 with me as the President and another well-known disabled warrior: Maj. Gen. Ian Cardozo as the Vice President. Since setting up the NGO, we have assisted a large number of war disabled personnel and at the same time by participating in the Mumbai Marathon for the last 10 years consecutively, spread the message that disability is no bar for continuing to deal with challenges. Our Foundation is funded by donors, and we do not get any monetary assistance from the government.

Simultaneously with my setting up the War Wounded Foundation, my wife set up an NGO of her own, named Retired Defence Officers Wives Welfare Association (R-DOWWA), which runs free tuition classes for poor children in Panchkula and Chandigarh. They too depend on donors for financial support and get nothing from the government.

While my Foundation was still in its nascent stage, the then Chief of Army Staff, Gen NC Vij, requested me to set up a 'Think Tank' for the army, which met another passion of mine, viz. enhancement of studies in military strategies and connected areas and in international affairs. Thus, I became the Founder Director of the Centre for Land Warfare Studies (CLAWS). I left CLAWS after five years, but the institution is still going strong, and my worthy successors have added much to it.

When my wife and I formally started our ageing process, the above institutions, besides helping those for whom they were set up, acted as anchors for our own advancing lives. After one retires, one must continue to be productive and happy, besides being content and trying to give more to society and especially to the needy. Unless one is engaged in pursuits that suit one's talents and likings, merely living in a mundane manner is neither good for you or society, and consequently the nation. Luckily, for people with a military background, a well-planned and disciplined approach is easy to adopt, as the military teaches one not only how to be a good and effective soldier and leader, but also how to approach a life of dignity that helps others both materially and emotionally.

At this stage, let me list some of the important points one learnt in the military, without any elaboration, as they are self-explanatory, which help one to look at ageing in a positive light. These are:

- Respect everyone,
- Life is not always fair, but keep moving,
- Don't be afraid to fail often,
- Take calculated risks, and
- Never give up.

Health is perhaps the most important factor that needs to be dealt with methodically, as good health enables one not only to live a stress-less life, but also to be a better and helpful individual who can assist others. We constantly hear about positive thinking, cultivating a positive mind-set and being positive. Let's understand its meaning. Positive thinking means right thinking at every moment. We expect the best, visualize the best to happen, but we also accept the outcome, whatever it may be.

Maintaining a positive mentality and getting appropriate and adequate exercise must be considered as duties and one must keep at them consistently. Health, in my view requires four activities, which are exercise, nourishing food, adequate rest and adherence to a fixed schedule.

If one is fond of animals, keeping pets is good for general well-being and learning from their habits and absorbing the love that they give you. The best therapy when you are worrying about anything is pets; the more the better! Pets are as sensitive as members of the family. They have to be walked, exercised, bathed, groomed, trained, fed, pampered, scolded, loved and treated like your own babies.

In the fast pace of life today, we tend to ignore or pay less attention to our environment as well as nature in all its wondrous glory. The reasons are our various preoccupations and what is conversationally called the 'rat race'! As one grows older, one must find time for absorbing nature and doing one's bit to restore it to its glorious past. Once again, those from the military are better suited for respecting nature, on account of their postings to hills and dales and all types of terrain and climate and with our habitats as close to nature as possible. In addition, our military cantonments are 'cleaner and greener' and indeed the lungs of our cities. We need to keep our homes and streets too in the same manner as we age.

A few parting words may be in order. Most of us are ambitious in varying degrees and we compete with colleagues and peers during most of our working lives. However, when we enter the last stage of our life, we need to adopt cooperation as our 'mantra' and shed competition, as the latter creates stress, fear, jealousy and moves us away from happiness. Co-operation earns blessings and makes us successful. Success here is not about racing ahead and being Number One. Success is measured by our happiness, health, beautiful relationships and our achievements. Co-operation is natural for us, so let's live the natural way.

We must also see the reality of life, so that we cherish what we have, enjoy life to the fullest, but stay humble. One must not act superior on account of our age and talk down to others. One needs to appreciate that the way of nature is the way of life; go with its flow and live with equanimity. Success is not to have a life free of pitfalls and falls but success is to walk over your mistakes and go beyond every stage where your efforts were wasted looking forward to the next stage.

While we are still ageing or have entered our last stage of ageing, we should continue to perform to the best of our ability/capacity. We must always remember that our life is our journey to our destination; it should be at our speed, using our capacity, and on the basis of our values.

Ageing gracefully doesn't mean you have to wear your wrinkles with pride - instead, you need to do whatever is necessary to stride into your older years with confidence. If you feel energetic and youthful internally, then it needs to be channelled towards positivity and age must not be looked at as just a slowing down process. We need to separate the physical process of ageing from the attitude towards age.

I cannot resist adding a bit of advice, which is what an American author, Todd Henry has written in his book, *Die Empty*, which he explains as 'Don't carry inside you the best that you have. Always choose to die empty'. The meaning of this expression is twofold. Firstly, to share your knowledge for posterity; and secondly, deliver all the goodness that is within you before you leave!

6
AGEING GRACEFULLY, WITHOUT LINKING IT TO ECONOMIC AGEING

DEVAKI JAIN AND SHIVANGI GUPTA

The ageing experience cannot be separated from the circumstances in which you live - whether you are born in an income group that is capable of providing some well-being or you are amongst the very poor where not only health but food itself is a challenge and where the circumstances of your home are so crowded that it is impossible to have any kind of sanitation. So this has to be related to one's economic level, exposure to opportunity, the environment in which one lives, as well as one's social strata. Education is the third part of the ladder of steps in which one can locate an issue like, how one responds to ageing.

Further, there is an often unarticulated but extremely important factor in how you age and that is, heredity. For this, one needs to read the remarkable book by Siddhartha Mukherjee, *The Gene: An Intimate History*. So class, caste, genetics, history, all play a role in the experience of ageing. I would also add that unless one takes note of this bundle of factors, to merely give advice on how to age gracefully would not only be inappropriate but cruel.

Speaking of myself, while others notice that I am at the age of 87, still able to walk, think and write, it is not due to my own efforts. These were gifts that I received because of my genetic history. Not only from my father who lived up to the age of 100, but his sisters who were actually living in extremely stressful, highly economically deprived situations, in faraway villages which had very few health services, also lived up to their 90s.

His cousins, some of whom were really church mice in terms of economic opportunity also lived beyond 90, and their children which include a sister-in-law of mine for all that she may neglect, she is still alive at the age of 90+. And her sisters, even though they lost their husbands decades ago and are older than her, are still there with their full minds.

Deterioration in age can take place not only physically but also mentally and by and large one associates a high level of age with dementia but again, age without any of those vulnerabilities is also a genetic gift. One of the worst aspects of ageing can be physical infirmity. Again, if one is able to manage without that it is entirely a genetic gift.

As someone who is now 87 and is in many ways as strong and capable as she was say 10 years ago, it has been a question in my mind also, how is it that I am still in this shape and form? There is a bit of stumbling in the mind that I forget names and sometimes even episodes in my life. It worries me but then I jog myself and say you are 87, so you must expect some slip. But it is true that my limbs, my legs, my arms are not very different from what they were 10 years ago. I walk without a stick; I sleep alone in a bedroom as a part of a flat which is rented by my son. I do things for myself like bath, dress or pick up things.

How does this happen at the age of 87? Well again, the answer lies in genetics and nothing that I personally did. I have to confess that I never did any exercises most of my life. I did not know yoga exercise and I did not take regular walks, nor did I have regular multi-vitamin tablets. So again, I argue that what I am today, that is, relatively capable in mind and body at the age of 87 is a genetic gift. At this point I would like to retain the mind at least, even if the body begins to get feeble because a very humiliating experience for ageing people is any form of dementia or Alzheimer's disease. It is said that the person who is suffering from these ailments does not recognize what is happening to her or him. It does feel terrifying to think of oneself as incapable of remembering, recognizing and being self reliant. These three are still attributes that I continue to have.

Do I do anything to maintain them? No. No particular tablets but I am told that there are yoga practices that can ensure it is maintained, especially the mind. I am told that pranayama can be a great help if the mind is failing. But always having been a very undisciplined person, someone who did not have any particular regime, any particular diet, any particular methods for maintaining herself, to be able to come to some grips with a discipline and regimen at the age of 87 seems quite a challenge. On the other hand, one would like to have as much compassion and caring for elders who have this declining attribute.

Talking of personal history, we were seven children to my parents, and none of us suffered from any physical infirmity. Again a genetic gift! The hitch and the Achilles Heel in all this of course is economic well-being: there are people who have lived well and long without having this genetic gift, and that is usually related to having good nutrition, having access to health services and enough financial capability to pay for health services. It is also to have children and relatives who are caring and enable people to live good lives till they die.

It is important to take note of this proposition that I am making because we are still in a situation where widows by and large are ill-treated, and not fed except for the last piece of food in the household. So, if a woman from a relatively less economically capable class or household gets widowed at an early age, their whole lifestyle, and their capability to enjoy ageing is threatened. Emotional and physical stress and decay are too often their lot. Thus, one cannot give them any kind of advice or even offer a model on the usual basis of age, gender, and opportunity.

Role of Culture and Society

As we reach a new stage of life, it becomes necessary that our beliefs and actions realign to reflect not only the personal decisions and desires that define our past, but also the cultural norms and expectations assigned to that particular life stage. As culture and society have modernized across both recent and distant history, new opportunities have arisen for women. Unfortunately, though, the culturally prescribed norms and expectations assigned to the various stages of a woman's life have not always kept pace, leaving her to balance her traditional familiarity with a quest for modernity. What she wants to do is not always what she ought to do or what others expect her to do.

As the length of life and number and proportion of older persons increase in most industrialized and many developing nations, an important question becomes whether this ageing population will be accompanied by sustained health, an improving quality of life, and sufficient social and economic resources. The answer to this question lies partly in the ability of families and communities, as well as modern social, political, economic, and health service delivery systems, to provide optimal support to older persons.

Thus, ageing as a health phenomenon is again associated with social, economic and demographic factors. However, while all modern societies are committed to providing health and social services to their citizens, these systems are always unstable, guided by various policy formulations. An interesting example of a performing system is from Karnataka, India, where large numbers of Dental Schools, mostly in the private sector, have made oral healthcare more accessible for the older population.

The need for integration of old age care into the universal health system crops up repeatedly as a solution to complex healthcare issues in old age. Most of the care of older persons, in their last few days to months, takes place in hospitals or at home. However, for a minority of patients who have severe physical or cognitive disability, dying at home is not an option, as there may not be a family to take care or the family at some point of time fails to cope with the burden of care. Long term care for these people is a challenge for the health system and the number of such dependent persons is rising steadily with the decline in family support.

Ageing through the Feminist Lens

Different disciplines on ageing have different perspectives. However, one common perception is that lived experience is a confluence of history, culture, and most importantly the accumulation of the opportunities and constraints one has faced earlier in life. The book *Age Matters* by Toni M. Calasanti and Kathleen F. Selvin, explains that age pervades feminist thought as well as wider societal thinking. Classic feminist theory recognizes race, class, and gender as the primary organizing principles of power. The concept of ageing and age-relations has been ignored by feminists. In other words, traditional feminist theory does not consider how age relations structure the opportunities available to, or the expectations associated with being older vs. younger, and how those earlier life experiences are then compounded across the successive phases of life. In the analysis of older widows' lived experiences, Chambers used a life course framework to explain that grief is not as much about the discontinuity or disruption caused by the death of a spouse, as it is the continuity of one's previous self. On the other hand, *The Feminine Mystique* describes age as the source of inequality, which Betty Friedan could not recognize, until she herself experienced it throug age.

Gender Ageing

Even though many of the diseases or conditions common to later life are experienced by both men and women, the actual rates, trends, and specific types differ between the sexes. While some of these differences are the result of physiological differences, to fully understand ageing and health a gender perspective is required. Gender can be understood as the complex and differing pattern of roles, responsibilities, norms, values, freedoms, and limitations that defines what is thought of as "masculine"and "feminine" throughout the life course and which all play a role as determinants of ageing. On the other hand, men are more likely than women to avoid seeking medical help, at least until a disease has progressed. Further, men's life expectancy is shorter than that of women.

However, in most countries, the combination of various health and social factors result in a lower quality of life for women in later life. A study by the Harvard Medical School states that men's hearts age differently than that of women. As widowers, older men tend to be more isolated than women due to perceived lack of male skills in developing social and familial ties, as claimed by the report by the World Health Organisation.

Though men and women tend to age in a similar fashion, however before the age of 50, women age twice as fast as men. This is a finding of a study published in the *American Journal of Physical Anthropology*. However, given the advancement in technology, the anti-ageing health and medical products market is growing rapidly, in both industrialized and developing nations, thus masking the fact that women are aging and that entire industries have helped create a market for anti-ageing products.

There are of course many ideas and practices/prescriptions that are afloat on how to avoid further deterioration of anything in the mind or the body. I still think that some of the practices suggested by yoga are perhaps the best. In terms of medication, I think some of our traditional ideas are most valuable, for example, the use of turmeric, the use of fenugreek. Fenugreek is supposed to have an impact in terms of staggering if not holding back the onslaught of diabetes. Turmeric, not only as a disinfectant but as a barrier to disease, is also something I believe in: for coughs and sore throat, I still think that turmeric milk is a good idea. Masala chai also is a great chai, and so it goes with various prescriptions of food and drink coming from Ayurveda.

In conclusion, I come back to my original thesis that much of good health or bad health, much of the fact that we may have depleting diseases like diabetes or asthma etc. is genetic and we have to work hard between the ages of 40 and 50 when these genetic troubles begin, to avoid them.

7

Ageing as It Touches Your Life

Justice Sujata Manohar (Retd.)

Shakespeare with his renowned felicity of language, called life a stage, and urged: "Act well thy part and there all honour lies." The role you enact on this stage of life may change with age, but honour lies in playing the role well. Not everyone has the good fortune of living a long life. Those who have enjoyed a long life have learnt how to cope with the joys and sorrows of ageing – joys of playing with grandchildren and even great- grandchildren, the pleasure of seeing the success of one's children or success of a long-cherished project; and sorrows connected with health problems, loss of friends and dear ones, and at times the - financial or other difficulties faced by one's family.

But if you have played your part well, recognition will come as you grow older and your contribution to social well-being gets recognized. So ageing has its own rewards. It also has some inbuilt setbacks, particularly if medical problems set in or mental and physical faculties fade. An ability to cope with setbacks is at the heart of living a full life at any stage of life.

It is difficult for me to talk about my ageing because oddly enough, there has been so much to do that I did not have time to think about my age. So let me retrospect. I have enjoyed being a woman. It gives you freedom to enjoy and to participate in performing arts - music, dance, theatre, or other aesthetic pursuits such as doing Rangoli on festive occasions, decorating the house, experimenting with cuisine, and so on. Fortunately, men also participate in these creative activities more freely now. Also, there is nothing comparable to the joy of bringing up children. Right from childhood I had decided that I would lead a balanced life working outside and inside the home. I felt a little sorry for men who were denied a lot of such pleasures in concentrating on success in the outside world. And I felt equally sorry for women who could not look beyond their home and hearth. There is now an increasing realisation that both men and women need to participate in home and social life as well as in economic activities and public life. And I hope that the future society will be structured to give scope to both men and women to lead a balanced life.

What made me choose law as a career? In my family there was a tradition that one son would become a doctor and the other son would become a lawyer. That is how my father's elder brother Dr. R. T. Desai qualified as an ENT surgeon from London while my father qualified as a solicitor and as an advocate. My father became a top lawyer and, later, a judge of the Bombay High Court and Chief Justice of Gujarat High Court. We are 3 sisters. My youngest sister had a choice. She also decided to become a doctor. That is how, right from the beginning, it was decided that I would be a lawyer.

Let me touch briefly on my academic career as it affected my work, the way I was initially treated at the Bar and was later given recognition. In the SSC examination I stood 5th out of about 60,000 students in the then State of Bombay, and was first amongst girls, winning three scholarships and prizes of the Board including the prestigious Chatfield Prize and Dadabhal Naoroji Scholarship. Since I wanted to become a lawyer, it was necessary for me to take arts: I graduated with first class honors in Philosophy and Sanskrit. I had created a university record by winning 6 University scholarships and prizes including the S. G. Selby Memorial Prize, Gangabai Bhatt Scholarship and Venayakrao Jugonnathji Sunkersett Prize in Sanskrit in my Intermediate Arts examination.

I joined Lady Margaret Hall, Oxford and obtained an MA in philosophy, politics, and economics — a three-year course which

I was allowed to complete in 2 years. I qualified as a barrister from Lincoln's Inn, London, and returned to Bombay (as it was called then) in 1958. I joined the Bombay bar . In those days women who tried to practice law were not taken very seriously. They were considered incompetent and unsuitable to practice as lawyers. I have mentioned my academic background because I could not be accused of being incompetent. Nevertheless, it was quite difficult to get work for some time. However, I did ultimately manage to get reasonable work. This was the start of my working life and the beginning of the ageing process. During this period, I got married, ran my house and had three children. So life was full.

I was appointed as a judge of the Bombay High Court in 1978. Thus began the second stage of my working life. Was this the start of the ageing process? I had no time to think along these lines. I was the first woman to be so appointed. I realized that I must do well if women were to be considered in future for judgeship of the Bombay High Court. I believe that I have discharged my responsibility. There was of course the greater responsibility of doing justice impartially and in accordance with law to those who came before me. I discharged this important responsibility to the best of my ability without fear or favour, affection or ill will and in accordance with the Constitution and the laws — thus living up to my oath of office. I became the first woman Chief Justice of the Bombay High Court and then the Kerala High Court. In 1994 I was the second woman to be appointed to the Supreme Court of India. I retired in 1999.

I suppose one can say that the ageing process clearly starts with retirement. I retired from the Supreme Court at the age of 65. My husband and I expected to lead a quiet life with my doing occasional arbitrations and opinion work. In a sense, a professional never retires. The present Attorney General K. K. Venugopal, the former Attorney General Soli Sorabjee, and the eminent lawyer Fali Nariman are all in their 90s. I was appointed a member of the National Human Rights Commission soon after retirement. NHRC then was a very prestigious organization and was considered one of the best in the world. Justice J. S. Verma was then the Chairman. As a lawyer I had worked with many NGOs and women's organizations helping them with their legal problems and working with those who came to these organizations for legal help. This work had given me a lot of satisfaction. I was very happy to get an opportunity to make an even more effective contribution to social well-being by becoming a part of NHRC. My five years with NHRC were extremely rewarding. I was put in charge of matters relating to women and children in addition to looking at my share of the various complaints relating to violations of Human Rights which came before the Commission. With the cooperation of the Institute of Social Science, and with the help of 11 NGOs working in the field we brought out a major publication dealing with trafficking of women and children in India, the areas from where the victims were entrapped by gangs of traffickers, the centres where the trafficked victims were taken, the reasons which led to trafficking, interviews with victims of trafficking and even some traffickers. It was action research which was accompanied by many rescue operations. It was a unique study which attracted attention throughout the world.

The Vishakha judgment of Justice Verma to which I was a party had aroused international interest. I was asked by the United Nations to talk to judges in Africa and in the Caribbean about enforcement of International Human Rights treaties through domestic courts. I was also invited by the UN High Commissioner for Human Rights as one of the 17 judges from around the world to advise on requesting enforcement of Human Rights by domestic courts without impinging on the jurisdiction of domestic governments. There were other similar interesting assignments in addition to the heavy workload of the Commission. When I retired at the age of 70 from the Commission I had worked to my full capacity without any concession to age.

I'm afraid I have not finally retired as yet. Stephen Leacock, the Canadian humourist has written a delightful essay on "When men retire". He talks about the man obsessed about his health after retirement who spends his time looking for medicines, standard or exotic. Then there is the man who wants to catch up with life at Las Vegas and Paris and Monte Carlo. He ends up in hospital. Obviously, there are several interesting ways of planning one's retirement. There is nothing in the essay about when women retire. Maybe they never do. After my retirement from the National Human Rights Commission, I have led a busy life, hearing cases for arbitration, both national and international, as well as writing opinions. My health has sustained this workload. Apart from swallowing several pills in the morning and at night, I do what I can to discharge my responsibilities to my family and in respect of my work. I am happy that my family has done so well. With advancing age, one tires a little more easily and needs breaks. That apart, life is as enjoyable or as worrisome as ever.

Descartes, the famous 17th century French philosopher, talked about the meaning of life. He sums it up in one sentence, "cogito ergo sum" (I think, therefore I am). Perhaps one can add to this summation, "I think and feel and care, therefore I am." Age is a process which the body undergoes. What matters is life and how you lead it. If you think and feel and care, you are as old or as young as you want to be.

8
My Journey to Senectitude
Tahir Mahmood

In 1996, while I had another five years to go before becoming a senior citizen by legal definition, the government put on my shoulders the onerous responsibility of chairing the National Minorities Commission (NCM). Soon I convened a meeting of all national commissions of the time in the NCM Conference Hall. Among the dignitaries present there were two great law brains of the country VR Krishna Iyer and LM Singvi. It was there that I had first Mohini Giri, President VV Giri's daughter-in-law, who was then chairing the National Commission for Women. Soon we had become comrades-in-arms. The two chairs we occupied were no beds of roses. Our ways of discharging our respective obligations to the two disadvantaged sections of the citizenry earned us both bouquets and brickbats. Our shared experiences of those three hectic years laid the foundation of a long- term fraternal relationship between us. By the time sister Mohini demitted office in NCW she had already become a senior citizen, while on completing my term in NCM I had to wait for some more time to get that grey- hair distinction.

I had taken up the NCM assignment on deputation from Delhi University where I had been teaching law since 1974. Before returning there I went on a long sabbatical to update myself in the legal disciplines of my interest. Resumption of work at the university coincided with my elevation to senior citizenship by law. In 2003, three years before retiring from DU, I put in my papers there and moved to Amity, an upcoming educational hub that was destined to become Asia's largest private university. The atmosphere there, very different from Delhi University, was exceptionally congenial and gave a boost to my academic and extramural activities. Continuing there till date, I have enjoyed seventeen years of high respect and deep affection at the Amity campus in Noida, and it eminently shows that a peaceful work atmosphere coupled with intellectual freedom is a precious factor for a happy advancement towards senectitude.

My life-companion, Naz, had worked for nearly three decades in a leading business organization of the country specializing in beauty culture and dermatology. She had joined them in a lower rank but by her hard work eventually rose to occupy one of their topmost administrative positions. By a strange coincidence she voluntarily bade farewell to them at the same time when I left Delhi University. After an intervening sojourn with her own independent work in the same field, she decided to give it up and devote all her time to social and humanitarian service. At this juncture, sister Mohini Giri once again entered the arena of my life. Naz joined her renowned institution, the Guild of Service, and is continuing to work for it in an honorary capacity. What had begun in 1996 between me and sister Mohini as comradeship in national service thus became a family bonding.

Before earning the tag of senior citizenship, my life had been most active at two particular junctures in my career – first in my mid-forties when I had played a lead role in building *vox populi* in favour of the apex court's *Shah Bano* judgment relating to divorced women's rights; and then in my late-fifties when I worked as the NCM Chair in rather unfavourable political surroundings. But no less active, indeed, have been my years even after earning the distinction of being a senior citizen.

During the decade of Dr. Manmohan Sigh's captaincy of the nation since 2004 I served, at his behest, on two other national commissions – i.e., on the National Commission for Religious and Linguistic Minorities, headed by the octogenarian Ranganath Misra, a former Chief Justice of the Supreme Court; and on the

18th Law Commission of India, chaired by another apex court judge, AR Laxmanan. Working with these top judicial brains was a lifetime experience, contributing a lot to my carefree years of unabated activism. Both are no more alive, but I keep reminiscing about our joint ventures to serve the nation.

I had my higher legal education in England and as a seeker after knowledge have travelled to country after country across the globe. My foreign travels have in fact been most frequent and vibrant after crossing my mid-sixties, but never tired me so as to affect my academic output. On the contrary, watching the world beyond India and being in the company of renowned scholars and intellectuals all over the world abundantly enriched my knowledge and also impacted my thought process.

In my sixty-fourth year I had published my thematic autobiography, *Amid Gods and Lords*, truthfully describing my experiences with religion and law, and the votaries of the two social-control mechanisms. The extremely resentful response to it from my kith and kin kept me mentally disturbed for a while, but I decided to drown my anguish from these unexpected quarters into new academic work and spent the next fifteen years in unprecedented activism, without letting my growing age dampen my spirits. Since 2008, I have published a dozen new books, including a revised and updated edition of my autobiography, raising the total number of my published works to forty-two. The higher courts of India have honoured me by citing my works in numerous judgments, and this has indeed been a rejuvenating factor for me.

Despite my extensive studies and research, and a life full of vast experiences gained worldwide, my family and friends expected me to remain an orthodox person not only subscribing to the outmoded interpretations of religious precepts but also translating them into my lifestyle and conduct. Happily, I did not oblige them - though deviation from orthodoxy and tradition cost me the love of my elders and relatives and turned friends into opponents. I have since faced the worst of foes among those who should have been the best of friends, witnessed protégés turning into bitter enemies, and encountered devils among those masquerading as angels. But I always remained what I was and have firmly stuck to my views.

The most annoying paradox I have witnessed all my life is a gross violation of human rights in the name of religion. Followers of various faith traditions claim existence of binding human rights injunctions in their holy books. I have no quarrel with them but stare at such claims with disbelief when I find the most conspicuous violations of human rights taking place in the name of religion - rights to life, dignity, equality before law, personal liberty, freedom of speech, gender and juvenile justice, all being denied on religious grounds. My respect for religion gets a jolt also when I see human rights being sacrificed on the altar of superstitions and blind religious beliefs.

In my opinion, if religion has to be retained in human society it has to be as a cementing and not as a dividing force. If religions must create a rift between man and man, I will be happy without any religion. Justice Krishna Iyer had once observed that "Religion cannot be wished away or wiped out, but must be humanized and weaned from cannibalistic habits. Comity of denominations, not a zoo of savage faiths, must be the governing code of religious pluralism in the human world." This exhortation of the great jurist-judge sounds to me like my own conscience call. I hate religious polemics and cannot accept the claim of any religion to have a monopoly on spiritual truth.

Ever since I became the master of my views, I have put humanism above both religion and law. Against the inhumanities inherent in the traditional interpretations of laws supposed to be divine, I have been protesting in writing and by word of mouth. I believe that neither religion nor law is an end in itself – both are means to achieve justice, fair play, and humane solutions to all our societal and individual problems. I am of the opinion that law must override religion, and vice versa, where this ensures a more humane behaviour. If by ignoring a law, religious or worldly, I can do justice to someone, or deal with a human being in a more humane manner, i will not mind doing it; and have in fact done so on many occasions in my life.

On the whole, I have lived my post-sixty years more actively than before. Looking back at my bygone years, I realize that among the most important factors that enabled me to age gracefully were my decision to turn vegetarian at about the time of becoming a senior citizen, and my continuous preoccupation with academic work. At this mature stage of my life, I keep reminiscing about every moment of my past life and feel that I have nothing to be repentant about and no reason for any feeling of depravity. Continuing to work hard, for much longer hours than many of those much younger to me, I still have passion for reading and writing. I remain a student, learning new things minute by minute. At the same time, I am a humble teacher always trying to pass on to others all that I know or have experienced.

And, unknown to many, I have been a poet and singer. Since my early adolescent days, I have been composing Urdu poetry, and singing it in private gatherings. Unusual for an academic, this extraordinary hobby has been a strong energy-booster for me. Let me conclude this brief story of my journey to senectitutde with a few extracts from one of my poems:

Yeh din mujhe har sal ye deta ha manadi,
Qudrat ne ghari umr ki eik aur ghata di.
Sadshukr ke bharpur nibhaya isey maein ne,
Ye zindagi bahton ne jo bas yun hi ganwa di.
Kuch log mujhe dil se yahan piyar hain kartey
Bas eik isi ehsaas ne kuchh umar barha di
Hoshiyar ke haim kaam abhi aur bhi leney
Aflaak se kis ney hai mujhe aaj nida di.

Translation:

This day every year gives me a warning:
Nature has reduced life by another innings.
Thank God I have lived it so fruitfully.
The life that many others just live aimlessly;
Some souls here love me from heart's core
This feeling advances my life a bit more.
Beware! You must work more before you sleep.
This call from the skies on my mind I always keep.

This poem was written by me on Teacher's Day nineteen years ago. Signing this write-up for sister Mohini's book on this year's Teachers' Day, I feel exactly the same.

9

TEN TENETS OF ENDURING LONGEVITY

DR. RAGHUNATH MASHELKAR

People know me as a scientist. But they also know me and call me a dangerous optimist. My essay will reflect both these sides.

Two people reach sixty years every second both in the developing and developed world. But the challenges that the elders face are different in the developing and the developed world. The developed world became rich first and then it became old. We in the developing world are going to be old first and then become rich. The challenge has become even bigger after the Coronavirus pandemic. The pandemic has destroyed lives and livelihoods. The poor are the worst hit. And we have further added to the pool of the poor. In just over 100 days, around 100 million families plummetted from poverty to extreme poverty. Being poor is a challenge. But being poor and old is a bigger challenge.

And that is exactly the challenge that our International Longevity Centre is trying to address.

I have been privileged to be the President of the International Longevity Centre-India (ILC-I) for over a decade now. This is a not-for-profit organisation working for the cause of population ageing. ILC-I believes in 'Celebrating Age and Creating a Society for all Ages'. It has been working actively with a direct interface with senior citizens. Serving ILC-I has been a great learning curve for me.

We must provide opportunities for the elderly, where they can add value, to the society as well as to themselves. ILC-I started a programme where the senior citizens can add value by promoting values in the education of young children. As we know, we badly require value-based education today.

Here the elderly, with their accumulated wisdom and understanding of the world, interact with school children, imparting to them precious values which they might miss in their education in school and indeed even at home. And this is a win-win situation. The children acquire precious values, and the elders feel younger in the company of the young.

The present pandemic has posed a particularly serious challenge for the elderly. This is a section of the population that is most vulnerable to the corona virus and as a result, it has restricted the elderly to the confines of their homes, just to ensure their safety. Such a forced isolation has impacted the mental, physical, and emotional health of the elderly. Not being able to go out and exercise, not being able to meet friends and relatives or socialise, all this has been traumatic for the seniors. ILC-I addressed this particular concern so that the elders could cope with this challenging situation and stay active and healthy. If not physically connected, the elders can remain digitally connected, but for that they have to be digitally literate. ILC-I created a Mobile Literacy Training for senior citizens. It became so popular that we had to resort to new models of training of trainers to satisfy the demand. During the pandemic, it was modified to make it into a virtual training programme. Special videos on how to use various social media communication apps like Google Duo were incorporated, as was the very important app devised by the Government of India - the Arogya Setu app. The entire focus was on maintaining and enhancing the mental and physical well-being of the elderly in these trying times.

How can we make high technology work for the poor and old and that too especially under Indian conditions? In order to trigger innovation in this domain, through my personal donation, ILC-I created an award 10 years ago in the name of my mother. It was called Anjani Mashelkar Inclusive Innovation Award. All the awardees have done a remarkable job in using high technology work for the poor. What were the common characteristics of their innovations? They all are extremely affordable, an essential requirement for the old and the poor. But they belong to what I call 'affordable excellence'. This meant that they were low-cost, but at the same time highest in quality. Secondly, they were designed for Indian conditions, using non-invasive technologies which do not require any specialised trained manpower, are very easy to operate, and user-friendly. These innovations range from non-invasive and affordable blood haemoglobin detectors, portable ECG's, diabetic neuropathy, and breast cancer detection.

Here are some interesting illustrations. In India, a woman is diagnosed with breast cancer every four minutes and its incidence is on the rise in both rural and urban India. Many victims are poor and old. Early detection is the best way to improve breast cancer outcomes and survival rates. Mihir Shah learnt that over 90% of women in the developing world did not have access to any mechanism of early detection of breast cancer. To fill this gap, he came up with the iBreastExam, an early screening device for breast cancer. iBreastExam uses innovative sensor and material technology combined with software computing to accurately identify cancerous lesions and tumours. It is a portable, radiation-free and non-invasive US FDA-approved device ensuring that the screenings are safe, pain-free and private. They have also proposed an innovative pay-per-use model – instead of targeting direct sales –which allows doctors in every corner of the country to start screening women for breast cancer at a cost that is less than Rs 100 per scan, as against mammography, which is very expensive, besides being painful. A safe, affordable and radiation-free breast exam can be conducted in the convenience of a community health center or the home. iBreastExam is commercially market-cleared by US FDA, CE mark and eight other regulatory bodies in Southeast Asia, Latin America and Middle East. In 2017, GE Healthcare announced a distribution partnership with UE LifeSciences to bring iBreastExam to women in 25 countries.

Let us look at another problem that the old have. With nearly 30 million people suffering from heart ailments, India is unfortunately known as the heart disease capital of the world. Heart attacks are also notoriously difficult to detect. 'Sanket' electrocardiogram (ECG) device created by Rahul Rustogi, is a disruptive high-tech innovative solution for personal cardiac care. It is a credit card-sized heart monitor, which acts like a portable ECG machine, making it possible to monitor the heart condition, making it as simple as monitoring body temperature. The high-tech 12-lead ECG recorder connects to a smartphone wirelessly, and displays and records ECG graphs on a smartphone. The ECG report can be shared instantly with a doctor via e-mail, Bluetooth, or even via WhatsApp. The affordable device marks a dramatic shift in the way we approach cardiac care, doing away with expensive ECG machines, distant hospitals and laboratories, and skilled technicians.

Another problem of the old and poor, is severe diabetes. Diabetic neuropathy damages nerves in the legs and feet of diabetic patients. These foot infections are the single largest reason for hospital admissions of diabetic patients. Every year about 25% percent of diabetics develop ulcer-related complications that ultimately result in amputation. In this backdrop, Dr. Jairaj Chintamani made a simple observation. He found that extremely neurosensitive, weight-bearing human feet are able to maintain a huge mass of living tissue. But the majority of human and animal feet possess dead, insensitive, and calloused tissue. This observation inspired him to create a non-invasive device, Diasense, that allows a physician to measure the neuropathy and pinpoint high-risk ulcer-prone zones in the feet, thereby allowing the physician to initiate preventive measures. This helps prevent the formation of foot ulcers and gangrene development, potentially helping the patient avoid an amputation. This high-tech device offers a unique and individualised solution that uses sensors that run on a software to predict the possible ulcers with almost 90% accuracy. The device offers a non-invasive procedure, user-friendly software interface, report generation in less than five minutes, and no consumables, hazardous materials or byproducts are used or generated. In addition, it is easy to operate, and anyone can be trained to do so. It could also prove useful for patient management for other diseases that involve nerve damage, such as leprosy and multiple sclerosis.

Another challenge of the old is vision-loss due to eye diseases. Shyam Vasudev found that more than 90% of eye care equipment was not affordable for hospitals in India – they were imported, not portable, and needed a lot of power and expertise. It would take 3-4 hours to perform all the tests and require some eye drops to be administered by a nurse. Shyam decided to do change the game. Thus, 3nethra was born – an intelligent, portable, non-invasive, non-mydriatic, low-cost device that helps in pre-screening of five major eye diseases, namely, cataract, diabetic retina, glaucoma, and cornea & refractive index, with powerful inbuilt auto-detection software. The 3nethra is a digital fundus camera, equipped with an efficient workflow to capture high-resolution images of the human eye through a quick focus mechanism that reduces the examination time. It costs one sixth of the current cost of collective pre-screening devices and can be operated by a minimally-trained operator. The solution has a value proposition for everyone in the entire eye care value chain, namely, the elderly blind, doctors, eye hospitals, rural entrepreneurs, and pharmaceutical companies.

Another challenge for the poor and the old and is iron-deficiency anaemia – which also afflicts women, who make up half of those who suffer from anaemia.

Anaemia can be diagnosed and treated relatively easily; often patient monitoring turns out to be the most difficult task. Unfortunately, some patients may live at a distance of up to 15 miles from a primary health centre. Myshkin Ingawale invented a handheld, non-invasive device to measure blood Hb, christened ToucHB. This portable, battery-operated device can produce an on-the-spot reading, without a prick. The patient simply has to place the finger in the clip or probe, and the readings are available within 60 seconds!

It works using optical technique photoplethysmography (PPG), where light of different wavelengths is shone through skin tissue. This helps in understanding the concentration of Hb in the tissue. The user need not possess any special skills to use this device. Since there is no need for needles, lancets, micro-cuvettes, blotting paper etc., recurring costs are limited to the expense for batteries, and no bio-waste is generated. In addition to haemoglobin, ToucHB also measures oxygen saturation, temperature and pulse rate – all for INR 10, just a small fraction of the cost of current tests!

ToucHb is a real game changer and a boon for millions of poor old people around the world, who suffer from undiagnosed and therefore untreated anaemia.

These five are examples of Indovations, meaning innovations created for Indian conditions by our very own young Indian scientists and technologists for the poor and the old that we at ILC-I have not only given awards for, but also promoted, and not just in India, but globally – as these innovations offer 'affordable excellence', the whole world can be a market for them.

A lot of people ask me as to how come even at the age of 77, you are so extraordinarily active, so positive? Here is something that tells you the secret.

You might say these are crazy dreams. Can a country, which has so many deprived, so many people below the poverty line, so many illiterates, really do it? What gives me the confidence that it can happen?

This confidence comes to me because of the images of a little boy, who in the late fifties studied under the streetlights and went barefoot to the school until he was twelve years old. A little boy, who struggled to have two meals a day; a little boy who was to leave studies in 1960 after his matriculation, in spite of securing a position in the top thirty in Maharashtra State SSC Board, because his poor widowed mother could not support his education. This boy was helped by this gracious Indian society. He rose to be the President of Indian Science Congress at the dawn of the new millennium. If this miracle can happen to an Indian, given an opportunity, it can happen most certainly to every Indian in the coming millenium. In the concluding words of my Presidential Address on "My Dream of India in the 21st Century" atthe 86th Indian Science Congress on 3 January 2000 in Pune:

"Next century will be the Century of Mind; and India will have the legitimate right to lead. Next century will belong to India. I believe this will happen as this dawn of the new millennium turns into a morning, and what a glorious morning would it be for my India." Late Prime Minister Atal Behari Vajpayee was then presiding over the inaugural function, with an audience of around 5,000 scientists.

The answer as to why, even at 77, I am super active is that I am a self-appointed Chief Inspiration Officer. My job is to spread happiness and hope. And I am able to do that because I follow some mantras. Let me conclude by sharing with you those ten mantras, which will create enduring longevity with a longevity mindset.

First, you can't help getting older but you don't have to feel old. To me age is just a number. You are as old as you feel.

Second, age is mind over matter. If you don't mind, it doesn't matter.

Third, you must do everything possible to make sure that you're adding life to your years as you add years to your life. And you can do this if you live life fully, and forget about your age.

Fourth, remember that you don't stop laughing when you grow old; rather, you grow old when you stop laughing. Similarly, you don't stop playing when you grow old; rather, you grow old when you stop playing. Also, you don't stop thinking and creating when you grow old; rather, you grow old when you stop thinking and creating. So: keep on thinking and creating, laughing, and playing - and you will live long.

Fifth, your date of birth is not decided by you, but your date of departure from this earth is largely in your hands, and that day will depend upon how you live, physically, mentally and spiritually. If you maintain the highest standards in each of these, physically by exercising, mentally by meditating; but also spiritually by continuously exploring the beauty of the inner world, having a sense of meaning and purpose, loving and being loved, tapping into inner peace and joy, being of service to others, bringing comfort to someone feeling lonely and anxious, you will age gracefully.

Sixth, those who love deeply and give graciously never grow old. They may die of old age, but they die young. So: keep on loving, keep on giving; and this giving can take several forms.

Seventh, even an old tree can spring new buds. Ideas and creativity are not the prerogative of the young. Let me explain by taking the scientific community as an example, since I am a scientist. And I have seen that Prof Hildebrand wrote his book, on diffusiòn in solids, when he was celebrating his 100th birthday. Sir G I Taylor wrote a single-author paper in *Journal of Fluid Mechanics* on the stability of soap films, when he was 93. Professor John Goodenough got the Nobel Prize when he was 97, but as he approaches his century, he still keeps active in his research. Coming nearer home, here is my Guru, Bharat Ratna awardee Prof C N R Rao. He is 86 now. But he is still in his laboratory every morning. His enthusiasm for research is the same as it was when he was in his twenties. And he produces the same number of research papers as he did 10 years ago. My favourite is Keki Gharda. He has donated so generously to ILC-I over the past several years. We are beholden to him, because we have survived and succeeded in serving the cause of the humanity mainly because of him. He just celebrated his 91st birthday. Keki Gharda is an innovator par excellence. He built his entire billion-dollar enterprise, Gharda Chemicals, based on his research and innovation. To him, innovation is a way of life. Even at the age of 91, I find that he behaves like a 19 year-old, and any time you meet him, he's talking about the next breakthrough technology of his dreams. He is donating all the wealth that he has created to a foundation, so that not just conceptualising but actualising a world-class breakthrough of technologies can happen. One of them that I am familiar with will surprise the world. So, it just doesn't matter how old you are, all that you need is a purpose, perseverance and passion.

Eighth, you are never too old to have a new dream or set a new goal. When Dr. Narendra Jadhav, the then VC of what was at the time called Pune University, opened the Ph D program for the senior citizens, the response from them was amazing.

Ninth, remember the quality of life has improved vastly. So today's sixty is yesterday's fifty. So just subtract ten years of your life from your real age, and you will not only feel younger but live longer.

And, finally, my tenth Mantra. There is no limit to human endurance, there is no limit to human achievement, there is no limit to human imagination, excepting the limits you put on yourself.

Yuichiro Miura is the oldest person in the world to ever climb the summit of Mount Everest – at the age of 80. He first set the record in 2003 at the age of 70, but reclaimed the record – after other people had beaten it – when he was 80 years old in 2013.

This leads me to an important point. If you do not put any limit on what you can achieve, then what it means is that you have to say to yourself that your best is yet to come no matter how old you are. And for this I have a simple mantra for you. It doesn't matter whether you are 60 or 70 or 80 or 90. Make it a practice that every morning when you get up, you say to yourself that your best is yet to come and maybe today will be the day when the best will come. You will have a new lease of life and you will live long, and you will live a life that is full of happiness, contentment, full of peace and full of tranquillity.

10

AGEING, BEGINNING OF A NEW LIFE

DR. ARMAITY S. DESAI

The Context: Early Childhood and Youth Experiences of Ageing in the Extended Family

When does one really begin ageing? Although arbitrary ages are assigned such as 60 or 65, the actual feel of one's ageing is different for each one of us. I could not imagine I was already 60 when I was that age, nor at 65. It was only when my body started to give me hints that I realised then that, perhaps, I was beginning to feel my age. Since the process of evolution of our physical self on a life continuum flags us change, we are hardly conscious of the fact that we have begun to age. I do not think that I really and truly began to feel my age and its limitations till I was 80, so full and busy was my life.

Growing up I saw my grandparents ageing so gracefully that I did not see it as a handicapping condition. My maternal grandmother was often sitting up comfortably propped up on her big bed embroidering saree borders and taking snuff! She and my aunt, her youngest daughter, dressed every evening and went for a walk in the nearby maidan. Sometimes, they visited us climbing a hill slope where our building was situated 3 floors above. My maternal grandfather cycled around Mumbai doing his errands till he was 75 and had to be stopped by my mother, not because of age, but because he did not take any notice of the fact that the traffic in Mumbai had changed much since he began cycling in his youth! He would put out his left hand and make a left turn from an inner lane and would be thrown off by the oncoming traffic.

He really thought the road belonged to him! Once, he, my aunt, my brother and I (adolescents then), went to see off my parents at the railway station. When we came out of the station, evening traffic was heavy on the busy arterial road. My grandfather felt we were his responsibility so he nonchalantly went to the middle of the road and stood with both his arms out like a traffic policeman, with traffic coming to a screeching stop, and he herded his flock to safety across the road! Moreover, till a very late age, he carried his cycle on his shoulder up a flight of steps hewn in the hill, to his house at the top, and climbed ladders to pick his jasmine flowers growing on a creeper. He was indomitable.

My paternal grandfather was the head priest in a Parsiagiary (fire temple) and occasionally visited us. At 80 he laid down his office, visited my father in his office and told him he was retiring to Navsari, his hometown, to die there. Not much later he expired. His wife, my grandmother, lived till 95. Even as she was ageing, she kept herself busy spinning very fine yarn from sheep's wool to make the Kasti (sacred thread) worn by Parsis and bestowed at a ceremony initiating them to the religion at ages 7 to 9. Thus, my perception of ageing was very positive, with none of the trauma expressed in the literature. I, on my part, decided I should live only till 60, it seemed to me, as a school girl, quite enough for a life span! My friend, who is no more, and I decided we would age gracefully, not dyeing our hair and allowing it to turn grey slowly!

The above description is the context of ageing in which I grew up and saw it as a natural and normal process. None of my grandparents were ill for long and though my maternal grandmother had problems towards the end at the age of 98, I was out of India at the time, and did not see her end.

Reality of Ageing and Death: Facing It in Immediate Family in Adulthood

In my own family, my father lived to 80 and my mother till 91. Both suffered fractures of the leg towards the end of their lives and were at home with me so that I could make them as comfortable as possible. That has been the greatest plus point of India, that the elderly were sheltered for the most part in their own family. Among the Parsis, those who could not live with a family had old age homes to care for them. None were on the streets. I recall an American social work educator who came to my house for dinner and saw my mother nearing age 90 being given special soft food easier for her to chew. He said enviously how we looked after our aged in our own homes, individualising their needs, compared to his own country, where they entered special senior citizens living arrangements. I recall also at a Christmas dinner, to which I was invited by my Dean of Students at the University of Chicago, School of Social Service Administration, declaring to some of her colleagues who were present that she would not like to go to a senior citizens home as she would no longer hear children's voices. In contrast, when I took my mother for an evening outing in the Tata Institute campus (where I was Director) in a wheelchair, the young children of families residing in the campus, playing in groups, would flock to her and surround her calling her grandmother! Almost like an Indian extended family!

It is not as if pain does not visit us, and the reality of ageing and death are met face to face. Within 10 days of my shifting my parents to the Tata Institute campus, my father fell and fractured his leg while closing the front door. He was hospitalised locally, and I had to coordinate staying with him in the hospital and managing the Institute. Parsi families are small. My brother worked in Bangalore and there was no extended family to support except my mother's sister, who came and looked after my mother while I was in the hospital. A retired professor, who lived on the campus as he was married to a professor teaching in the Institute and lived in the faculty quarters, sat with my father till I could go home, have a bath and lunch and come back refreshed. My father never recovered fully and walked with the aid of a walker. Subsequently, he had a stroke and died within a year and a half after moving to the campus. It was a severe blow for me as I was very close to him. He was a very warm and sensitive human being, and I felt his loss greatly. It all happened in less than 2 years of my new job. It was also a great emotional blow to my mother who became somewhat disoriented and needed full time care but did not want anyone sleeping in her room. She fell at night and had a fracture, and my hospital routines started again. Remarkably, she fully recovered. However, within a short time, she fell again and had another fracture from which she recovered; but pain from a pin that had shifted due to soft bones, never left her and I had to get a wheelchair and round the clock care. To ensure that she would not be lonely, I was with her for lunch and as soon as I came home in the evening, I sat with her in the family drawing room before bath and then dinner together. She sat after dinner while I worked on the files and then retired to bed while I stood by her bedside to wish her goodnight. Sometimes she had problems at night and her caregiver would wake me up to comfort her. She lived seven years after my Father and passed away at home one afternoon after I had helped with her sponge bath and started her lunch. She enjoyed the lovely mangoes my brother had left us and, soon after, death came visiting.

During this period, my brother had a cancer operation at the Tata Memorial Hospital, and I was shunting again between the hospital and my job. I felt a complete orphan with no family except my brother. Later he shifted to Bangalore, where he founded Titan Industries (making digital watches(and Tanishq (making state of the art jewellery) for the Tata group of companies. Though younger than me, he suffered from heart problems for which I had to rush to Bangalore; but by that time I had retired and was not torn between job and patient care. After being with him in his illnesses and seeing him well again, he subsequently contracted dengue and passed away. He and I were very close, and his death shattered me as it came so unexpectedly, when I was groping with my own ageing body and back pain resulting in bedrest. He was my great support emotionally and I had no immediate relatives left. Although I have my sister-in-law, she is busy with her work life, and my niece and nephew are both settled out of India. So I have been very much on my own in my old age and learned to be self-sufficient emotionally and in day-to-day living. Changing circumstances, as one ages, demand resilience and the capacity to face and handle events even as one is ageing and having to bear the loss of loved ones.

Retirement and a New Life Forward

I retired at 65 as Chairperson, University Grants Commission, in 1999, having worked earlier as Director, Tata Institute of Social Sciences (November 1982 to February 1995) and as Principal, College of Social Work (affiliated to the University of Mumbai (Nirmala Niketan, June 1957 to October 1982). Having held responsible positions in my jobs and satisfaction with a very fulfilling career, retirement was a welcome change. It felt like a newly acquired freedom from the chains of a job which required one's full attention and commitment, besides doing tasks which one enjoyed as much as doing those required by one's position, although not as enjoyable. With retirement I was free to do what I wanted and free to refuse anything I was not likely to enjoy. I was freed from routines and decided that one thing different would be getting up as per my body clock and not dictated by my timings for work. I returned after 16 years, barring vacations, to live in the flat that had been always my home from age 5, having spent 12 years in the Tata Institute campus and a little over 4 years in Delhi. The first thing I did, even in anticipation of my retirement, was to start to redo my home so as to live comfortably in my old age. I had been living there since I was 5 years old and by 65 it certainly needed redoing. Besides retiling floors, wiring and painting, I redid my old-style bathrooms and kitchen. I had given away my parents' beautifully carved drawing room furniture to my brother so that his children could inherit them, and in its place my brother gifted me new furniture he designed and had made in Bangalore to go with the rest of my parents' old furniture. Comfort is essential as we age, and its design suited my ageing. I had also acquired two female full time domestic helpers while at the Tata Institute, who had continued to be with me in Delhi when I was appointed Chairperson of the University Grants Commission. As in Tata Institute so also in Delhi, they took over the management of the house, leaving me totally free to immerse myself in my new job while they explored all the resources needed to cook meals and to establish the household routines. Subsequently, when I retired and moved to Mumbai back to my home, they ran the house while freeing me for the various activities I undertook on retirement. Now that I am eighty-six, one has retired but the other is still with me. The bonus is that in view of my failing health, she takes considerable responsibility for the running of the house. It is essential that for single ageing women living without family support in the home, a dependable domestic help or a paid caregiver is absolutely essential. When you have recruited them in the best of times, they are a major support in the worst of times.

Do What Gives Most Satisfaction

I look back now aged 86 with satisfaction, not only at the three jobs I held at the College of Social Work affiliated to the University of Mumbai, Tata Institute of Social Sciences, both in Mumbai, and the University Grants Commission in Delhi; but also at the very active years I spent after retirement from age 65 to well over 80, when I had to start gradually withdrawing on grounds of health. This was also a gradual process over a period of 3 years. I still have four NGO responsibilities as Trustee/Executive Committee Member as they do not wish me to resign, but I am able to work with them digitally as I cannot participate physically due to a painful back condition. On retirement and return to Mumbai, I decided that I would now prefer to give what I had acquired in experience on a voluntary basis and not seek any projects with financial arrangements that tie me down, except those that would not consume all my time, and that too very few and far between. I was Board member of two universities, a Trustee/Executive council member of several NGOs, and spent more time now on writing and publishing and speaking assignments and travel for meetings in India and abroad. I cannot name all the activities but I will choose those that were challenging and stimulated me.

An all-engrossing activity was a UGC programme to develop women's leadership among faculty and administration in the universities and colleges. The programme had 3 types of workshops: a foundation workshop to develop sensitivity and awareness of what kept women back from such positions as department heads, directors of examination or affiliated colleges, physical education, vice chancellors, registrars and such leadership roles in academia. Five manuals on five different topics were developed for trainers to use by women's studies experts, who were our main resource persons, many of whom were retired persons. The training was for five days and training methods suitable for adult learners were used. Those completing the basic workshop could move to specific skill-based training on topics related to management. Manuals were developed by our own experts, who were also our resource persons and knew the context for developing manuals in these subjects. Two topics were completed in 6 days. The third workshop was on the training of trainers and manuals were developed for training skills. Initially the same resource persons undertook the training; but to encompass the vast expanse of India with many colleges and universities, the workshops for training of trainers provided well trained persons to undertake the workshops.

The workshops were established in their allotted region by regional heads who implemented them in various locations in their region in either a university or a college, with participants deputed by Vice Chancellors from the universities and colleges in their region, making a batch of 25 to 30 participants. The change in the attitude of the women was phenomenal. Coming with doubts to the first foundational workshops as to how such a workshop could benefit them, they left with a changed perspective of themselves and their worth as women leaders, free of age-old conceptions of patriarchal views on women's capacities for leadership. The programme covered institutions from Leh in Ladakh in the North to Rameshwaram in Tamil Nadu in the South, and from the western borders of Rajasthan to the East in Mizoram, Arunachal Pradesh, and Meghalaya, not to leave out territories such as the Andamans, Male and Pondicherry. Some outcomes included women achieving status as department heads, director of examinations, registrar and 3 vice chancellors. Resource persons were assigned to each region, and they proctored the workshops helping the newly trained women trainers. Keeping up the quality of the workshops was of prime concern. Everyone worked for the programme in a voluntary capacity to organise the workshops. Payment was only given to those who produced manuals and to regional heads, resource persons and trainers who guided the workshop. As the chair of the committee on this UGC project, I travelled to many workshops in different parts of India, which gave me an opportunity to understand and learn from the feedback as every workshop was evaluated, both orally and on paper. Unfortunately, 10 years after its operation, the UGC, in its patriarchal wisdom, closed down the programme. Sadly, all subsequent chairs have been males, and none of them restored it. Although some scattered workshops are being given, there is no monitoring and expansion of the programme.

Another time-consuming, but a most fulfilling activity, was the ChildLine Foundation of India. The programme was started as a field action project of the Tata Institute of Social Sciences in the early nineties to answer calls and provide intervention for street children and other children in need with an easy-to-recall number 1098. Such field action projects were started by the Institute which could demonstrate new or innovative areas of service or method of service delivery. The spirit behind this project was a member of the Faculty, Jeroo Billimoria, who had experienced the problems street children faced and often received phone calls from them from public phones. As Director of the Institute, she came to see me with the desire to start the activity. I agreed but asked her to use existing facilities such as institutions for children and NGOs, rather than spend money on bricks and mortar. Space was provided by the Municipal Corporation of Mumbai in one of its schools for a small rent. The special number was allotted by the Telecom Ministry after representation to them. A grant was obtained from the Sir Dorabji Tata Trust to commence the project and cooperation with the British Council ultimately led to cooperation with ChildLine in the UK and the establishment of an international association of child lines by Jeroo Billimoria.

Without any furniture, sitting on the floor on bedsheets, social workers were recruited, and the service started and calls began to pour in as the social workers contacted street children and information on the service rolled out. Children's calls were for various services such as need for shelter, desire to return home as they had run away from various parts of the country, and even neighbouring states such as Nepal and Bangladesh; rescue of children from trafficking and child labour, often working in deplorable conditions; child marriage; fear during examinations; health needs including hospitalisation -especially wanted by street children, and countless other needs. The project was based on child rights and, hence, no attempt was made to force any child to do anything the child did not want, such as institutional care or return home.

Within a couple of years of the project demonstrating such call-based outreach of children in need, Maneka Gandhi came forward as Minister for Women and Children to take over the project funded by the Ministry and to expand it to other cities and in time to over 600 districts in India to cover the needs of rural children, with strategies evolved suitable to rural outreach. The country was divided into regions with regional offices and some measure of decentralisation. The programme was fully supported at the state level by the Central Government. States like Kerala wanted more call centres and hence willingly supported the additional centres. The support came from several hundred NGOs who were funded to carry out ChildLine activities in addition to their own programme. Not a rupee was spent in construction activity. Only the ChildLine Offices in Mumbai and the state regional offices were hired. A major expense was hiring trained social workers, and some money was spent on children's direct needs. Individual call centres were later replaced with centralised regional call centre facilities which managed calls and directed only cases where intervention was required to the appropriate ChildLine agency. The project ran as a public-private partnership with the Central Governmen, with a joint Board of ChildLine trustees, under the Secretary of the Ministry of Women and Child Development as chair, and a couple of senior officers of the Ministry besides the original ChildLine Trustees. As a trustee, I took responsibility for all matters related to the social work activities and development of the programme, and Mr. Nawshir Mirza, also a Trustee and a Chartered Accountant, looked after the finances.

In the meantime, Jeroo Billimoria had married a Dutch national and moved to Amsterdam, The Netherlands. She had already laid foundations for setting up an international organisation while in ChildLine, arranging a conference with representatives from other countries. With the help of the London ChildLine, she established an international organisation with its headquarters in Amsterdam. She not only brought in existing organisations but also set about starting such services in the developing countries of Asia, Africa, and South America. The Indian model of ChildLine was preferred as an outreach programme, whereas, the European model only received calls, counselled children and if they needed continuing service, they were referred to an existing service. With the paucity of such referral services for children in developing countries, the Indian model of physically reaching out to the children was preferred. Jeroo insisted, during the foundational days, that I come on the Board of ChildLine International. This gave me opportunity to contribute to another developing organisation. In time, The Government had been facing problems with some NGOs in India who had not rendered an account of funds sanctioned and hence the Ministry imposed a

Bond on Trustees of all NGOs that they would be responsible for paying back the funds to the Ministry. This was not possible for persons like me as the revenue and capital expenditure annually was mounting towards one crore and I had to resign along with some other Trustees including M. Mirza. We tried to explain to them that ChildLine India Foundation was unlike other NGOs as it was a public-private partnership and the Secretary was the Chairperson of the Foundation; but this seemed to evade the government, which made sweeping rules without understanding implications. I was very sorry to leave an organisation after possibly a decade and a half of activity, which I had been a part of since its inception and helped nurture, but changes in Government policy resulted in my departure. Still in touch with some of its senior staff, I am gratified to see its development upon the foundations we had laid.

A third one with which I have continued as my resignation was not accepted, but to which I respond to all papers digitally, since I cannot be present at meetings, is The Foundation for Excellence and Access, situated in New Delhi, which provides students at the rock bottom of the economic ladder access the best possible organizations, to acquire degrees of their choice. Coming from families of casual workers, crafts workers, casual agricultural workers and similar lower level and mostly unskilled occupations, these students- despite their deprived backgrounds and poor access to education, score high percentages in Class 12 and seek finances for their higher education. The scholarship is unlike the bare minimum provided by government and some non-government organisations because it fully covers all expenses and additionally provides a programme of life skills. Its students have graduated from IITs, medical colleges, and other well-paying courses, as also those who went in for basic sciences and social sciences. It is extremely satisfying to see the difference it has made in the lives of these students. Government keeps talking of upskilling. Our experience shows the capacity of these youngsters to perform when finances are not a matter of concern and anxiety, and in the end to pull themselves and their families out of poverty.

A fourth intellectually satisfying experience is my membership of the Parsi Zoroastrian Foundation for the Preservation of Vulnerable Heritage (PARZOR Foundation) in Delhi as the Coordinator for Research on Population and Health of the Parsis of India, a fast-declining community demographically. In collaboration with a Faculty at the Tata Institute, three research projects were undertaken on the family, youth and ageing. All three were published by Sage Publications and included a fourth volume with researched articles. All four were edited by a colleague at the Institute, Professor Shalini Bharat and myself for publication.

Besides my affiliation with NGOs, I had opportunity to work with government institutions such as the Union Public Service Commission on two of their policy making committees, with the University Grants Commission on some Committees, and International Child Helpline on their Board. Besides the challenges inherent in developing future looking policies, being connected to institutions which were being newly established in their foundational years such as Pratham, ChildLine India Foundation, International Child Helpline and Ambedkar University were challenging and stimulating experiences. Being invited to the Board of the Tata Institute of Social Sciences had a lot of emotional sentiment for me as it was my alma mater, having graduated from it in 1957, worked part-time at a faculty there in 1962-63 while employed full-time at the College of Social Work affiliated to Mumbai University (Nirmala Niketan); returning to it in November 1982 as its Director, and ending up on the Board during my retirement. It was a full circle and an extremely satisfying happening in my life.

With the freedom that came with retirement, I at last had time to write. Besides contributions to edited books and journals, I had time to accept invitations to speak at various forums and sadly also at the passing away of persons with whom I had been professionally associated, for whom public memorial meetings were held. While domestically I had a well-organised household with considerable stability in my domestic help, I had an old aunt who lived close by and the only remaining member of her generation in the extended family, to be looked after, and a male cousin who needed supportive help after my aunt passed away. I had to persuade him to go back to Navsari to his sister and wind up and transfer his finances as well as sell the flat and allocate the money as per my aunt's will. All these were very new experiences for me even as I was ageing, but they taught me a whole load of new things to prepare for my own end of life. One can never stop learning.

Conclusion

I am grateful for the experiences granted me after my retirement. I never felt cut off professionally and at the same time could undertake activities of my choice and work at my pace. My roots are in Mumbai and life has been kind to me, although now, at 86, I have a few non-lifethreatening health problems – mainly a painful back induced by sitting at the computer for long hours after retirement, and trigger fingers due to holding mobiles. These are the hazards induced by technology for older persons. I am able to adjust to my new normal which means staying home for most part of the day in bed and doing all I can from it on my mobile, including staying in touch with my group of professional associates, and emails for various tasks including managing my finances, insurance and some legal matters pending and a house in Navasari to be sold and the proceeds shared with all the legatees. Life chores are never ending. Solve one problem and another is at your door waiting to enter. But one has to take it philosophically as it comes, even though these can be irritants. For instance, partial deafness handicaps me in listening to interesting programmes on TV or using the phone. Fortunately, my eyesight was saved by successful operations for cataract which allows me to remain in contact with people digitally. One finds a way around one's problem. Until the pandemic descended on us, I had the pleasure of friends visiting, students long forgotten asking to visit or get in touch on WhatsApp, the pleasure of friends giving parties in my own home for my birthday and celebrating it on WhatsApp in a unique way. During the pandemic when we could not meet, friends offered to shop for me, my young physiotherapists helped me to learn how to shop and pay online with credit cards that I never used in my working life nor while I was still mobile! I learnt to work on the computer, a new skill, only after retirement when I did not have the luxury of a secretariat to do my typing. Similarly, I picked up working on both the computer and mobile through non-formal means, getting help as needed. It is never too late to learn. Ageing does not mean loss of one's faculties. It has been comforting to have so many people still in my life, even when mostly confined to the bed, filling a vacuum caused by having no immediate family living with me and only my sister-in-law in Mumbai and my brother's two children living abroad. While modern means of communication has kept the small family closer together, they are not there to undertake any responsibilities. It is made up by these life-long ties that grew especially in interaction during one's career. I am grateful for the very fulfilling life I had during my career years and after retirement, and wish that many who read it have also experienced a satisfying life.

11
Shaleenta se Jivan Jina
Aruna Dalmia

श्रीजी

शालीनता से जीवन जीना

मेरी प्रिय बहिन श्रीमती मोहिनी गिरी जी ने कहा कि इस उपर्युक्त विषय पर अपने कुछ अनुभव शेयर करूं । विषय तो बहुत ही समय के अनुसार उपयुक्त है ।

जीवन तो सभी को प्राप्त होता है और जो आया है वह जाएगा भी अपने निर्धारित समय से , लेकिन इस जीवन को कैसे जीया जाए ताकि वह शालीनता बनी रहे । बहुत समय व्यतीत हो जाता है यह सीखने में कि क्या ठीक रहा क्या नहीं तब परिपक्वता आती है और उसी को ध्यान में रखते हुए अपने जीवन की शैली को उसी के अनुसार चलाने में ही grace है ।

मैंने तो यही सीखा है और समझा भी है कि यह मानव शरीर प्रभु की सृष्टि की सबसे सुन्दर कृति है और वह इसके द्वारा न जाने क्या - क्या करवाता रहता है । जीवन की यात्रा के भूत काल को मैं नहीं दोहराना चाहूंगी लेकिन जब से यह समझ में आया है कि मैं तो मात्र एक यंत्र हूं और उसने जब जैसे नचाया वह करती चली गई । जब सोचती हूं कि यह सब कैसे हुआ और किसने किया तो यही समझ में आया कि तू तो मात्र यंत्र एवं दृष्टा है और उसी का कार्य कर रही है तभी तो जीवन के इस तट पर शालीनता बनी हुई है । कुछ पंक्तियां याद आई वो उत्कृष्ट कर रही हूं । प्रभु की कृपा के आश्रित रहने से न आयु ने अपना असर किया न परिस्थितियों ने :

हुआ समर्पण प्रभु चरणों में जो कुछ सब में था मेरा आनन्द ही आनन्द ।

मिटे सभी संकल्प , हो गया उनमें ही सारा अवसान |
कौन , कहां , कैसे , क्या करता रहा न इसका भी कुछ मान ।।
जब तक अपनी मौज मौज थी तब तक कभी न थी कुछ मौज ।
मौज बने जब से वे मेरे , तब से सदा मौज ही मौज ।।

– अरुणा डालमिया

English Translation

My dearest sister Mohini Giri ji has asked me to write a few lines about my experience of ageing, an issue that is indeed very relevant in the present-day world.

Everyone has a birth. Everyone who comes must go. Everyone's time of departure is already fixed. However, the vital question is, how to live this life with dignity and honour? It takes a long time to learn what is right and what is not right. After that experience we live a life of dignity and grace.

I have always learnt and understood that the human body is God's most beautiful creation and he makes us to do multifarious activities through this body.

I do not want to repeat my journey of earlier days but however, since the day I understood that I was only an instrument of God, I have followed Him to His command.

When I think how and who has done all the work of my earlier years and I realize all that He has made me do, has given me a life of dignity and peace today. I remember a few lines and I would like to quote them.

They convey that if you take the shelter of God, age then can not determine the meaning of your life.

This is dedicated to the feet of the lord.

May peace and peace prevail!

All my wishes merged into Him.

Who, where, how and what I do I have no idea
Till such time I was innocent and lacking in understanding;
I knew nothing……
The day God became my understanding, since then it is grace and grace

Hua samarpan prabhu charanon mein jo kuchh sab mein tha mera aanand hee aanand!
Mittee sabhee sankalp ho gaya unamen hee saara avasaan!
Kaun kahaan kaise kya karata raha na isaka bhee kuchh maan!
Jab tak apanee mauj mauj thee tab tak kabhee na thee kuchh mauj!
Mauj bane jab se vah mere tab se sada mauj hee mauj!

12
Growing with Sewa
Ela R. Bhatt

Ghelubhai, an aged acquaintance asked me, “How come in your old age you are still so busy with your work?”

I said, “Why are you asking me? Go and ask the old!”

However, this was some years ago when I was 80. Today, if someone asks me, I may be able to appreciate that as a good question. How come? Because about a year ago, someone asked me to name the year SEWA (Self Employed Women’s Association) was founded. I could not remember the date. A week later, I forgot to give an important message to my son! A few days ago, while telling a story about Kavi Narsinh Mehta to my grandson, I forgot the name of the great poet!

The frequent bouts of forgetfulness continue, and I realize I am ageing. I have been a prey to Chikungunia ever since 2013. Physical weakness pervades ever since.

Oh, All right! Fine! After all, Ageing, old age, or senior years is but a continuum of our life.

It was Ramesh, my classmate, who opened my eyes to the world. It was 1949, and I was a shy and studious university student, who admired Ramesh from a distance. He was a fearless, handsome student leader who was collecting primary data on slum families for independent India’s first Census of 1951, and he invited me to join him. Learning about “how the other half lives” was a liberating experience, and it made a deep impression on me. Ramesh was hardly ever on the scene with me later in my public life—he was a private man, and we were partners in life.

His insight and analysis were critical in helping me come up with unconventional solutions to India's problems.

Fast forward to the future and facing the loss of a loved one. My husband Ramesh left this world so suddenly that I was left with a massive guilt in my conscience that I did not serve him enough. He suffered from a weak heart during his late fifties. My friend Anandlakshmi gave me a book named *Living, Dying* written by two highly acclaimed medical doctors, who were both practising medicine and teaching it. From reading the book I learnt that death and disease have no connection. Both are independent of each other. That is a lesson I learnt and took to heart so strongly that I came out of that terrible feeling of guilt. Now I am not afraid of any disease, not even corona. Death? I'm ready for it any time. I believe, God will keep me here till he wants work from me in the other dimension.

So, I believe if our story must be told, we must also speak of our life, our work, our purpose in life and our growth. When we women sit down to tell the stories of other women's lives, they are inevitably long and convoluted. Because stories of women are invariably bound together with the story of their family and their community. It is almost never just about her life, the growth, turmoil, joys, and sorrows. It always includes a host of others. My story is intertwined as it is with thousands of SE sisters. We grew up together. Without my SEWA *behens* I think I have no story.

Having met thousands of poor self-employed women from across the country, the plaint I heard in 1986 from a frail, shrunken woman, while visiting a small village in Bankura district in Bengal summarizes most of their lives. She had said, "*Kaaj naahi, kaaj kori maroo*," meaning "I have no (paid) work, the grind of (unpaid) work is killing me". These words speak of the life of every working poor woman in India. Among the poor, throughout the country every woman works, throughout her life. Work is central to poor people's lives. Therefore, I chose to build our Labour Union. In SEWA Union we have approached the question of work in several ways, which has given us an insight into how our society, through its legal, political, social, and economic systems, views and organizes work. We have struggled to make the work of the self-employed not only recognized as work but appreciated, celebrated, and marketed. The poor face struggles of being recognized at various levels, from the law, the employers, the government, policy makers, and scholars. We at Sewa learnt that the struggle needs to be carried on at all levels. This is the path we have walked for 40 years. The hardest I have faced is the educated middle class mindset.

Mubinaben is a 70 year-old beedi roller from Ahmedabad. She got married at the age of 17. Her husband used to earn a living by repairing cycles, which earned him 50 to 70 rupees per month. Mubinaben rolled beedis at home, to earn some money, while she looked after her family, which, over the years included seven children (four girls and three boys). As expenses mounted, Mubinaben took up other sundry work. By the time their fifth child was born, her husband had become addicted to alcohol. Whatever he earned thereafter was spent on his drinking addiction. Mubinaben, struggled to bring up her children, trying to earn enough with whatever work she could get. As the children grew older, they took up some work, along with their studies. The boys studied up to the 7th and 8th, but her younger daughter finished school and completed a year-long teacher training course. Mubinaben bought a sewing machine and taught her daughter tailoring skills, making shirts and sari petticoats. When the children were old enough, she got them married and settled. All along, she continued her work of rolling beedis, making about a thousand per day. During the communal riots, their slum was also under attack. Putting the memory and dark days of the riots behind them, the Muslim and Hindu families live in harmony now. She prays that her children never have to go through the difficulties she has had to face in life. Mubinaben has been associated with SEWA for 40 years, and has also served as an elected member on the Board of Directors of SEWA bank. Among her neighbours, she has been raising awareness about

SEWA and its work. Her life has been full of sorrow, but she feels happy about being in SEWA. She now wants her grandchildren to study well in good schools.

Since our total membership consists of working poor women (a third of whom are Dalits, and another third of whom are Muslim), SEWA members are always so severely hit by the communal riots that it is a milestone in all our narrations. They become the primary targets of systematic and vicious attacks — rape, assault, murder, arson, and plunder. Wave after wave of violence results in hundreds being killed, leaving behind widows and orphans. The fact that we tried to help create communal harmony, sometimes brought the rioting right to my doorstep.

In 1981, during a communal clash sparked by reserved medical seats, I had publicly taken a stand in favour of the Dalits, as many of our Sewa members belonged to the Dalit community. Many upper-caste students felt that as a Brahmin, my sympathies should have been with them, not the Dalits. While the poor were happy about my support, I raised the ire of many of my neighbours. They directed their anger toward me in the darkness of night. A band of young rioters gathered outside my home, pelting it with stones, breaking windows. Rioters were my own neighbours, old and young. It was the most traumatic experience that Ramesh and I had ever faced. We had to move out of our home for a few months. Our SEWA sisters, who all worked and laughed and sang together, were being pulled in different directions by their communities during riots. And yet as soon as they could, they were the first to venture out to each other's neighbourhoods to make sure their work sisters were safe. Translating our belief in communal harmony into our lived lives is always difficult. I have faced a lot of wrath from neighbours for the Muslim lady who has cooked and looked after me for many years. Mubina's story is, in many ways, my story too. While I was alienated from my neighbours and some relatives too, I found full support among SEWA sisters.

Balamma is a 70-year-old Agarbatti (incense sticks) roller who was born in Karnataka. From an early age she began to earn, cleaning vessels in houses, making flower garlands, working as a farm labourer. She got married at the age of 15 and came to Ahmedabad. Her husband was twice her age, thirty years old, who earned a daily wage of Rs1.15, but he was not very interested in working and was home most of the time. So, the responsibility of the household fell on Balamma's shoulders. They had three children. The older two realised how difficult things were for her, and to ease her burden began to work, bringing home three rupees fifty paise daily. Balamma rolled beedis at night, and agarbatti during the day. Despite her workload, she found time to make kites during the kite festival season in winter. All this earned her an income of Rs 30 to 50 daily and she managed the household with the money she and her sons earned. Balamma lived in Bapunagar, opposite Ajeet mills in the Bharat Govind chali. During the communal violence they had to face a lot of problems. Now the Hindu families have vacated their houses and relocated to Odhav area. But the families keep in touch and visit each other. Her husband passed away when she was sixty. Now she lives with her youngest son, and he takes good care of her. He doesn't earn much but tries to manage to make ends meet. Her daughter-in-law used to make agarbatti but now that machines are available for rolling agarbattis, hand rollers have lost the job that paid them at piece rates. It is very difficult to get any work, and inflation has hit them very hard. Balamma's whole life has been of struggle and hard work. She joined SEWA and used to attend meetings regularly. This helped her to resolve the problems she faced at work. Many other women who were introduced to SEWA by her and her daughters-in-law, are also members of SEWA now.

Like Balamma, there are millions of women whose existence is fundamental to the city's economy, and yet the city-dwellers do not care about the rampant exploitation of these workers. In fact, I became aware of their existence and their plight when Chandaben took me to the Sunday market, 'gujari', bazar on the riverbed, where the sellers and buyers were the urban poor. I met several women who were producer-vendors like her, carpenters, tinsmiths, quilt makers, idol makers, block printers, beedi rollers, loaders-unloaders, waste pickers. I found that every woman I talked to was in debt — not for lack of enterprise or hard work, but because she did not have any working capital and because she did not own her tools of production. I also learnt that since the income of poor women from any one type of work is usually not enough to make ends meet, they must have several income-earning occupations. In fact, 80 percent of SEWA members then were illiterate, engaged in multiple types of work. The unique problems of SEWA members made us look for unique solutions and their perennial debt led us to start the SEWA Cooperative Bank. From the beginning, our bank's emphasis has been on savings first as a self discipline.

Radha Rani is a very cheerful person with a positive perception of life, and does not sound like a 72-year-old lady. She is very modern and politically up-to-date, and loves to talk about her past. She was a garment stitcher who has been associated with SEWA for the past 25 to 30 years, and fondly remembers committed SEWA workers Zaitunben and Madhuben from her younger days. Later she also used to operate Amber Charkha and make khadi yarn along with her young daughters. Radhaben was born in Madhya Pradesh in a small mohalla near Indore called Toda. Radhaben was just 10 years old when her parents died. Her Uncle and Aunt got her married when she was 11. Her husband was 7or 8 years elder to her, and he worked in a textile mill in Ahmedabad in the night shift. She had learnt stitching and cutting for garments from her aunt. When she came to Ahmedabad, after marriage, she had ample time and so she asked her husband to get her a sewing machine. She started to stitch petticoats and earn Rs. 10/- for a dozen. Since she had to take care of the house and children, she could not devote much time to stitching, yet she managed some small savings so that she could buy her own small house. According to her a lot has changed in her life since her early childhood. People do not expect anything from each other, there is nothing to wait for or long for. The value of money has also lessened. She recalls the days when she bought gold from Manekchowk for Rs. 100 per 10gms. And today her grandchildren spend Rs. 20/- per day on snacks! People earlier on were truthful, did not flaunt their wealth, and food was pure and un- adulterated. And today weddings are far too ostentatious and too much money is lavished on the events. According to her, the money spent should be given to the bride to help her to start a new life. She is nostalgic about the past, when discrimination was far less. She laughs and says "*Ab mein par-nani ban gayee hun... aab mujhe par nikal aaye hai, mujhe toh udna hai*....(I am a great grandmother now, so I am ready to fly.)

Radhaben reminds me of the millions of women who work from home, contributing to the national economy, but their hard work is not counted. The livelihoods of millions of such people are not perceived as "work" and therefore it remains uncounted, unrecorded, unprotected, and unaddressed by the nation. They remain conveniently "invisible" to policy makers, statisticians, and theoreticians. Dividing the economy into formal and informal sectors is artificial—it may make analysis easier, or facilitate administration, but it ultimately perpetuates poverty. People like Radhaben work for decades, from teenage to old age, and barely get a fraction of what they deserve. But their identity is so closely tied up with what they do, that they cannot think of not working, whatever their age may be. Even when they find themselves physically fatigued from working in the fields or housework, they will always keep busy, taking on tasks that do not require too much energy. To be living is to be working, is the mantra for most women who are poor.

Soniben Devshibhai Rabari, 67 hails from the village of Meghpar Lakhpat in Kutch, Gujarat. She has been a SEWA member for 28 years. There are eight people in her household and their occupation is animal husbandry. She says that in her youth she was energetic, no work seemed difficult to her as she could perform any task easily and efficiently and manage her household work with ease and speed. With age now, common tasks are tough to do and are time-consuming. She can manage to look after 2 or 3 cattle at the most, and sit down and do some embroidery work. She has hypertension, and gets medicine for it from the nearby town of Bhuj. She is not able to work with the same vigour as in her youth and this does create a bit of a tension with her family. But overall, she is grateful for the family support that she enjoys. What she really enjoys at this age is to come to SEWA for the Union meetings. Even at this age she is enthusiastic about SEWA's training programmes in Legal Literacy that build her self-confidence and is always on the lookout for some work that will bring an interactive conciliation meeting with the police, etc. She enjoys the respect that she has gained in and through SEWA. In her village she tries to solve issues because of the confidence she has gained from SEWA. This has given her a much-desired status in her home, in the neighbourhood, and in the village.

She knows it is her farming, cattle and embroidery that give her employment and livelihood. She welcomes technological advances that have made work and life easier, and help her to earn more money. Today she does not just sell her milk in the local market but at the dairy where she gets money as per the fat content in the milk. This has earned her more money.

Devalben Mamubhai Rabari, 76, also from Kutch, has been with Sewa for 26 years.

She has four sons, and one daughter. Her youngest son who is yet to be married lives with her. When she was young and felt fit and fine, any work looked easy to do, but not so any more. With age, she feels she cannot work in the field any more, so she does only household work, and that too, not as fast as she did once. Now she can manage 2 or 3 cattle and do some embroidery that she can do at leisure. Her grandchildren, instead of spending some time with her prefer to spend time on their phones. None of them are bothered to learn the traditional skills in embroidery.

Sonalben and Devalben repeatedly speak about doing embroidery and their wish to teach it to their granddaughters.

This reminds me of the struggle we had to revive embroidery in many parts of Gujarat, but these women living in desert villages had no time to themselves since they had to spend hours fetching water. To revive embroidery, we had to revive waterbodies in the village after a fight of seven years with theGovernment.

But it is **Hansiba**, the grand old matriarch of SEWA, from Radhanpur, with whom I had many long talks and from whom we all learnt so much. She was getting on in years and we were talking about old age - "ghadhpan" as it is called in Gujarati. She said, like people, embroidery stitches also attain ghadhpan and die out. (*Tanka pan ghardha thaye*). She knew many embroidery stitches which have slowly become extinct, and she was the only one living person who knew them. Her remark led us to quickly arrange workshops where other SEWA sisters learnt eight of the vanishing stitches from her and included them in their work to reach the market. SEWA set up a museum where we preserved old specimens of embroidery from all over Gujarat, donated by family members. Later a workshop of local craftsmen with international designers led to a new brand named 'Hansiba', which now has branches in Ahmedabad, Delhi, Bombay and the 'Hansiba' brand is also available at a boutique in New York. Hansiba's photo hangs in Islamabad's SEWA office, as she inspired the 'Sabah' brand in South Asia.

Hajira Begum, from Kupwara, SEWA Kashmir, says she feels no difference in her ability to work. She works at home, in the fields with as much energy and confidence as earlier. She still grinds all the spices at home. Life has become easier, but she feels that food that is made with labour tastes sweeter. Earlier families used to gather, laugh, and celebrate festivals together. Now mobile phones have taken children away. She wishes to see the whole village as one big family.

Aso Bano from Wahidpura, Gandharbal, Kashmir, shared her life experiences. She says earlier she had courage and energy though she lived in poverty. However, one person earned, he could support a family of ten then. Now even if ten people work, they cannot live well, there is no *barkat* (prosperity).

Stories of our SEWA sisters from Srinagar are similar in their tales of poverty and hardship. But added to that is their life being so filled with fear and insecurity and uncertainty about the future. It reminds me that whenever we visited any area that had been devastated by any disaster, the women asked us if we had brought any work for them. Work for women spells security, solace, and a healing process. I remember that in Kashmir, many decades ago, the All India Handloom and Handicrafts Board was one of the most active in the country, with its rich tradition of crafts of silver, wood, papier mâché and the carpet weaving and wool textiles and products as rich and aesthetically pleasing as the natural scenery. However, the craft traditions and crafts families have been hard hit in the last few years.

Shantaben Paulbhai Vankar, from Mehrav Petlad village, Anand district, 75, who has been with SEWA for 35 years, whom I remember especially from our long struggle for the legal rights of the tobacco workers to have Identity Cards issued by employers, is perhaps the most vocal about ageing. Only when asked how she feels in health, she mentions that her legs do ache, but she walks two kilometers every day. She can do most work that she did earlier, but feels tired after that. She still works from 8 am, and looks after 20 savings groups of SEWA, and still worries about recovery of loans given to SEWA sisters. "It was difficult to collect dues during lockdown, so my husband was surprised to see that some of the women came to my house to return the loan they had taken from SEWA bank. I told him it was because of my bond built over 35 years with SEWA." Her land had been usurped by her brother-in- law, and, knowing her obsession with land, her sons bought her a small plot. There was a time when she worked as a farm hand in tobacco fields: now her sons have become advocates and give legal advice to those very same tobacco field owners. But she lives simply as per the Gandhian philosophy.

She feels she is blessed because of the good wishes of so many sisters she has helped, doing seva, and being of service to others.

She took a 9-day computer training course which has enabled her to connect online to 4000 to 5000 SEWA sisters. She is able to supervise her farm and send reports to SEWA office because of her tablet. She knows that the network she has created will survive long after she has left the world. SEWA had given a voice and identity to countless women like her. When Hilary Clinton asked the SEWA women at a gathering in Ahmedabad if they were afraid of anyone, they answered that when SEWA is with them they fear no one, not the policemen, not the judges not even their fathers-in-law. Shantaben fears nothing, and she is at peace and does not ever feel like giving up. At 75 she earns her own living. "Old age is inevitable, whatever has been planned for us, we must abide by it", she says "Who can tell when a withered leaf will fall from a tree?" (*Paku panu kyare pade, kone khabar*).

Shanta, which means peace, was the original name given to a project to help the families of riot-hit victims. It was meant for widows who had been rendered helpless when their husbands were killed before their eyes in communal riots. For the orphaned boys and girls, the project, backed by the then Prime Minister Atal Bihari Vajpayee, was called "Hamare Bacche". The riot widows, both Hindu and Muslim, were trained to become self-sufficient with SEWA Vocational training which shared the same name as the feisty Shantaben. The name Shantaben resonates among us all as a symbol of resilience. Proudest among these is Shanta Paulbhai herself.

So, in the minds of our SEWA sisters, ageing is just the extrapolation of the lives we have led, looking after our loved ones, finding strength in solidarity and the courage to speak collectively for women, work and peace. We feel that the years are added to our life so that we can add life to the years of others. Age, therefore, is not a surprise.

To sum up, what has guided me in life and work are Gandhi's thoughts. His four major principles have guided my thinking.

One is simplicity, because we recognise that adding complexity is not progress.

The second is non-violence. Violence is fundamentally inconsistent with freedom.

The third is dignity of labour, sanctity of labour. Labour is the law of nature, and its violation is the central cause of the present economic muddle.

The fourth is human values—nothing that compromises a person's humanity is acceptable.

On these four cornerstones of simplicity, non-violence, sanctity of labour and human values — we were guided to build our India.

Next when I meet Ghelubhai, I will tell him, yes, I am ageing and working.

13
ART OF AGEING
FALI SAM NARIMAN

First – a few words about the person who prompted this piece. When Dr. Mohini Giri wrote to say that the Guild for Service was celebrating its Golden Jubilee and planned to bring out a publication that documented the *Art of Ageing "positively, productively and gracefully*" (as she put it) my first thought was that the person who was the most outstanding example of ageing "positively, productively and gracefully" was none other than the heart-and-soul of the Guild! (This thought had originated with my wife Bapsi, who like me was an ardent admirer of Mohini). Mohini had often reminded us of a sign that we had read decades ago, whilst passing through the International Airport at Copenhagen that said "The world is moving at 105,441 kilometres per hour. So KEEP UP!"

Mohini has been 'keeping-up' all her life – not for herself – but for weaker sections, helping not just in nation building but in contributing to a more gender-just society. Her sense of dedication and compassion are unrivalled.

Now, about AGEING. I am unfamiliar with the so-called "Art of Ageing". Let me say that I have just aged, helped along, by the way, by the marvels of modern-day-medicine! I am reminded of the story of Konrad Adenauer, the first Chancellor of the Federal Republic of Germany, who when approaching the age of ninety, succumbed to a heavy cold. His personal physician (unable to be of much help) had to put up with the chancellor's impatience:)I am not a magician. I can't make you young again," the harassed doctor protested. The Chancellor retorted, "I haven't asked you to: all I want is to go on getting older"! No, age did not bother me, at least not too much, till I was 87 or 88. Till then, I was doing most of the things that I was doing at the age of fifty – bearing in mind poet Arthur Clough's warning: "Thou …need'st not strive / Officiously to keep alive".

But good things don't last forever. I had to undergo triple-by-pass surgery in January 2018, after which everything changed. I became convinced at age 89 that ageing was no fun if there was no family care.

We Narimans are a very small family, but we do care for one another. My wife Bapsi and I were married for 67 years, before she left us in June 2020. She was extremely proud to be a member of the Guild. She was ailing for long, and yet took the most ample care of me (as I hope I did of her). Each one of our loyal staff, from my secretary upwards, looked after our welfare, and now continue to look after me. Our daughter Anaheeta who lives in Mumbai, but who had been visiting us very often took ample care of us, and now takes care of me. And our son Rohinton, who is amongst the busiest of persons in Delhi, has been taking excellent care of us (and now of me) as does his ever-charming and ever-caring wife Sanaya. But the most loving and affectionate of our "caretakers" had been (and they are now my chosen caretakers): our two grandchildren Nina & Khursheed who almost daily visited us (when Bapsi was alive) and now continue their daily visits to me.

All this family history – though extremely personal – is only to impress upon readers how deficient is our public health system, and what all of us should do about it. I have a simple cure: don't complain – turn inwards. Turn to your own family and they will help you. The older one gets, hospitals beckon more often than we would welcome. But public hospitals are like courts – you go to them not because you want to, but only because you have to!

I am a lawyer by profession and the main thing I have done and do (sometimes) is to practice my advocacy in Court: real, or virtual as during the Covid pandemic. I reveal this only because I firmly believe that the medical profession, despite all that is said against it, is the noblest profession of all. Fortunately, the medical practitioners that we Narimans have known were compassionate and highly admired.

So family care is what we all need. Pope John Paul II, the Polish Pope once said, "As the family goes, so goes the nation, and so goes the world we live in". Recent statistics show (as the *UN Report on Ageing* tells us) that older persons are taking over the world, and the very old are ageing much faster than they ever did! And surprisingly, the developing world like India is ageing even faster than the developed world!

Criticisms are levelled against governments, not just our government. but all governments people have had to put up with everywhere, as to how little is spent on health care. But I would have you know that there are three countries in the world, the most disparate in outlook, that are world champions in health care. Two of them are professedly capitalist, the other is diehard communist. Sweden, in the north of Europe, spends over eight percent of its GDP (Gross Domestic Product) on health, while the USA spends as much as 7.9 percent of its GDP on public health care. GDP, as readers are aware, is a monetary measure of the market value of the required goods and services produced in a specified period of time, often annual. The so-called welfare State of Mother INDIA spends a little over 1 percent of India's GDP on public health care. The other country, the only other country in South America that has remained communist for decades, spends as much as 7.9 per cent of its GDP on health. That country is the relatively small island nation of Cuba. And that is why Cubans, despite being deprived of the many modern amenities of life, would never give up their communist way of living, since the state looks after them even better than their own family does!

But in our own motherland, we do need organisations like the Guild for Service for taking care – and good souls like Mohini

Giri to help those in need of support. But if the family and - God forbid - even the Guild should turn their back on us, then the only option left is turn to God, in hope and with a prayer!

Is there a God? I believe there is. But many, even the spiritually-inclined, are not quite sure. I am reminded of the story that our late Prime Minister, Indira Gandhi always liked to tell (according to Pupul Jayakar, in her fascinating biography of the great philosopher and spiritualist, J. Krishnamurti). When the first astronauts (all Russians) on their return from outer space, called on First Secretary Khrushchev, then the most powerful man in the Soviet Union, and he asked them in confidence, "When you were up in the heavens, Comrades, did you see mysterious lights and strange beings? Did you see a great, mysterious white-bearded figure surrounded by light?" The astronauts, after a little hesitation, truthfully said, "Yes, Comrade Secretary, we did." Khrushchev's reply was, "Oh, I was afraid so." But Khrushchev sternly warned them, "This is between ourselves– comrades – do not tell a soul."

The astronauts then went around the world and were much feted with fanfares. When they visited the Pope, His Holiness took them into a room, and confidentially asked them, "My sons, when you were up there, did you see lights or did you come upon a vast figure with a white beard?" Remembering Comrade Khrushchev's warning, they replied, No, Father. We saw no lights, nor did we see a bearded figure". The Pope said, "Ah, my sons, I thought so. But on your soul don't tell this to anyone!"

In the West, the family has already broken up. Sons and daughters, and grandsons and granddaughters, have no time for their fathers or mothers, grandfathers or grandmothers. They are too busy eking out a living for themselves without much support or help. They age and go to seed, all on their own! More than 20 years ago, the Supreme Court of the United States decided on what was then regarded as a highly charged question in ultra-modern US society: whether grandparents have a right to see their grandchildren when a parent objects. Fifty years ago, the question would have sounded a bit absurd, almost farcical. Nine Judges of the US Supreme Court (six of them grandparents themselves), heard arguments from both sides before issuing a ruling rewriting American laws on grandparents' rights, a topic not covered by the Constitution of the United States of America. In an amicus brief filed in the US Supreme Court the American Association of Retired Persons – which then had over 30 million members – lent their weight to the aggrieved grandparents in support of 'visiting rights'. In one particular State in the US, Kentucky, the state's highest court had ordered visiting rights for a grandfather against the wishes of married parents who claimed he was 'overbearing and intrusive'! Here were first generation rights colliding with second generation freedoms. When the case reached the US Supreme Court, the Court was divided. Not a very encouraging advertisement for growing old. We in the Asian continent are fortunate that we have an inbuilt social support system.

Many years ago, when the Father of the Nation was alive, and I often wish that he was forever alive, a journalist asked him what he thought of western civilisation. Gandhiji tried to evade the question but the journalist persisted. All that the journalist got out of him was a laconic, "Well it's a good idea". Gandhiji was only being polite. What he actually wanted to say was, "It is an appalling idea. And the less we have of it in India the better". With all the advantages of educating the citizenry, television has brought western civilisation to our doorstep, and some families in India nowadays behave, quite often as do families in the West: All mind. All money. No heart.

But God or no God, television or no television, in this world of believing and doubting, and then doubting and not believing, what sticks out like a sore thumb is that humans, in spite of being wounded by "the slings and arrows of outrageous fortune", have a profound belief if not in God, at least in the rightness of things. Like when Lord Pethick Lawrence – a former Secretary of State for India and a distinguished member of the famous 1942 Cripps

Mission to India - wrote to Gandhiji, telling him the following tale: A Parson was attempting to console a farmer who was worried about something, and the Parson said, "Put your trust in Providence, my man". The farmer answered him angrily, "No, no. I have no trust in Providence. He lost me my pig two years ago. He let my house be burnt last year. He took away my wife last summer. No. I refuse to trust in Providence. But I will tell you that there is a power above Him, who will pull Him up if He goes too far!"

Intense belief in some Supreme Authority, howsoever remote, is the ultimate consolation for all our worldly and ageing woes. The reason why old age was venerated in the past when life expectancy was low, was because it was out of the ordinary. No longer. To be old now is to be part of a huge and ordinary multitude.

I conclude with a message which is not mine. And it is not about ageing but about its twin, caring. It is what a great and noble soul Mother Teresa said in her acceptance speech in Stockholm when awarded the Nobel Peace prize in February 1980. She mentioned that the right to live was the most universally fundamental of all human values. And she went on to recall an incident in Kolkata which showed how anxious were the poorest and the lowliest to protect the right to life, not for themselves alone, but also for others. She spoke simply and with compassion, as she always did, and I quote her exact words: "I had the most extraordinary experience with a Hindu family who had eight children. A gentlemen came to our house and said, "Mother Teresa, there is a family with eight children, and they have not eaten for so long. Do something." So I took some rice and went there immediately. And I saw the children, their eyes shining with hunger. I don't know if you have ever seen hunger. But I have seen it very often. And she [lady of the house] took the rice, she divided the rice, leaving some for her own family, and then she went out with the rest. When she came back, I asked her: 'Where did you go, what did you do?' And she gave me a very simple answer. 'They are hungry also.' What struck me most was that she knew. And who were they? A Muslim family, and she knew. I didn't take more rice that evening because I wanted them to enjoy the joy of sharing."

The joy of sharing is an intrinsic part of caring. Both Mahatma Gandhi and Mother Teresa had emphasized the need not just to universalise human values, but also to universalise respect for them.

Let me end this piece on ageing with one last true story: When doctors told Arthur ('Art') Buchwald early in 2006 that his kidneys had failed, the famous American humorist declined dialysis, and checked into a Washington, D. C. hospice to live out his final days. A few months later, "The Man Who Wouldn't Die" was still there, feeling good! Whilst in the hospice he even wrote a rollickingly funny book titled *Too Soon to say Goodbye*. But when you have to go, you have to go! With all his wit and humour, ill-health and age outwitted him. He passed on in January 2007 but not before alerting the New York Times to make sure that "No Head of State or Nobel prize winner dies on the same day as me"!

14

AGE AND AGEING ARE SO BEAUTIFUL!

DR. SHOVANA NARAYAN

"Didi! How does it feel to be 70 years old?" The question from a 15 year old student of mine amused me.

"Do you feel any different as to what you were when you were 10?", I asked gently.

"No," was her solemn reply.

I said, "I too don't feel any different from what I was when I was 50 or when I was 25 or when I was your age".

"How can you be so active and agile on stage at this age?" queried another student.

And the questions went back and forth. My students were online, celebrating my 70th birthday. Laughingly I asked, "Since I am 70 years old, why do you still call me Didi?"

"But we cannot even think of calling you anything else! You are one of us," they chorused. The bantering went on for some time. It emerged that they could not even think of calling me Guru Amma because I did not behave like an "Amma" which according to them meant a person who did not mingle, who did not joke, who did not pull their legs – who was 'not one of them'. That I was strict but yet I was their 'friend' made me closer to them. It was a revelation in human psychology.

How was I to know then, that very soon thereafter, I would be asked to pen down my thoughts on 'ageing'? So here I am sharing my latest experience with you, and how accustomed we are to preconceived notions! According to such a mind-set, with age, a person has to retire, look vacantly at space, keep forgetting, do nothing except to tell children and grandchildren what they ought to do and how it was during their young days! Society seems beset with negativity about ageing.

The question is whether, with increasing age, we stop living and whether age defines how one should behave; whether we were supposed to compartmentalise our thoughts and actions every decade, because we have reached a certain age.

Today, life expectancy has increased. Lifestyles are different. No longer are women confined to their homes. Women are busy with their careers. Agreed that there is a retirement age in some of the positions in certain jobs. However, the kind of interests a person has, ensures that the mind does not cease to function, and that the woman is alert and on the move.

As for me, my dance which is my breath, my soul, has always been there with me. While I loved my 'other part' of my being, namely academics that was later replaced by civil service, I have never felt stressed out. Perhaps this was ensured by my passionate involvement, dedication, and sincerity in both worlds. I have been the gainer for never did I suffer from stress. It also gave me a chance to grow and to learn with every new experience, each so varied, so different from the other! With each such experience, I stood benefited!

Let us see the positive sides of ageing. Time and age have brought in mellowness, increased patience, understanding and maturity. It has also helped in allowing one to see life differently from the time when we were teenagers, for now we are able to distance ourselves and see the incident in its proper perspective. Perspectives change with your mind's working, with your mood, level of maturity or immaturity, degree of patience, changing environment and varied experiences! We are beneficiaries of these because of our age, for life is all about continual growth and adaptation to new circumstances and challenges.

Had it not been for age, we would not have had the benefit of opening old albums and seeing ourselves as babies, as children, as students on the first day of school, the hesitancy and excitement writ large when first venturing out into the big world, as proud young students proudly displaying the gold medals pinned on our shirts, as young adolescents laughing over our silly hairdo of the sixties, the bell-bottom trousers that we had sported, of our wedding day, of our children and grandchildren. Had it not been for age, we would have missed the excitement of Neil Armstrong setting foot on the moon, or of seeing the ushering-in of the first colour television in our country. Are we not lucky to have lived through an age where we saw computers that were as big as a huge ball room? Tell a child of today and their eyes go round with disbelief, for today the computers can be hand-held! Imagine the romance in the expectation and excitement of booking a trunk call to your beloved, waiting impatiently for hours for the call to materialize, then to be able to hear his/her voice – and that too for 3 minutes! So much romance was hidden in those little actions of ours, very different from that of the 'instantaneous today'!

This reminds me of a question posed to me by a veteran author-journalist way back in the mid-eighties of the last century. He asked as to why we dancers - even in the latter quarter of the twentieth century - still performed to ancient mythological legends relating to Krishna or Shiva or Rama. In reply I asked him as to whether he did not see Krishna in today's child playing pranks like Krishna did? Whether he did not see a mother scolding her child as did Ma Yashoda? Whether he did not see the impatience with which even today a beloved waits for meeting her/his loved one as did Radha? Names could be different, circumstances could change, but the essential core of human emotions and human relationships has always remained constant. We then discussed how the moon and the moonlit night still remained symbols of romance, whatever be the age – in terms of time or in terms of physical ageing of the body.

There was one occasion when I had plunged into deep thought when I found that my joints were giving way. For a fleeting moment it crossed my mind that I had aged. In the next moment, a vista of beautiful experiences raced like a film through my mind as to how fortunate I had been that I was able to experience life's ageing process in all its hues. It also allowed me to dwell on how at a young age, the body needed a flurry of movements to fill in the sketches that we were drawing in space in the field of dance which, with increasing maturity, gives way to a lesser number of movements (in dance) for extra movements are constantly being replaced with the depth of emotion, grace and maturity of age and experience.

It is so natural to start wearing a new adornment called wrinkles that comes in the wake of increasing age. Happy are those who wear their wrinkles with pride for each crease has so much story to narrate, so much experience hidden behind it, so much laughter, tears and so many suns and moons it has seen. Another process is the gradual loss of body flexibility, which itself opens the door to another world of marvel as we with amazement see how the body adjusts itself to every new situation. It seems that there is a hidden message in it that we should keep learning and never allow ourselves to stagnate, mentally or physically. Allowing my body to stiffen naturally accepting it to be its own process, I have enjoyed allowing dance movements to be moulded into the limits of what the body allowed at differing points of time.

The learning curve never ends, for every moment brings with it a new experience. What remains and should remain with us is the culture of compassion, culture of inner journey, culture of deep thought, culture of learning, and culture of appreciation and acceptance.

Erikson's theory of psychosocial development maintains that self-acceptance is crucial for the attainment of integrity because lack of self-acceptance leads to despair and reduced wellbeing. Ageing lies in our minds for it is, as Dr. Jagdeesh Kumar says, "not the process of making you old and ugly, but ageing is the process of making you bold and beautiful"!

So why not accept age and the beautiful process of ageing? Why should we fight nature? One ages when the mind ceases to function, when one loses the passion of learning, of appreciation, of acceptance, when one kills the spirit of spontaneity and eagerness that lies within every person, when we stop laughing, when one settles into the doldrums of predictability and when one stops surprising one's own self. The power to make life beautiful at all ages lies in our own hands - each one of us can craft it. Each one is a fleeting moment in the passage of time. The sun sets only to rise again. The beautiful colourful panorama caused by the rising sun is as beautiful as that created by the setting sun – "a blaze of color – oranges, pearly pinks, vibrant purples..."!

"Each day is born with a sunrise and ends in a sunset, the same way we open our eyes to see the light, and close them to hear the dark. You have no control over how your story begins or ends. But by now, you should know that all things have an ending. Every spark returns to darkness. Every sound returns to silence. And every flower returns to sleep with the earth. The journey of the sun and moon is predictable. But yours is your ultimate ART." – Suzy Kassem

Life with its process of ageing is a beautiful 'art' where experiences add hidden dimensions. Our wrinkles are clouds in the sunset sky about which Tagore says, "Clouds come floating into my life, no longer to carry rain or usher storm, but to add color to my sunset sky."

An old pop song says:

You will never grow old
While there is love in your heart
Time may silver your brown black hair
As you sit in your old rocking chair
But with love in your heart
You will never grow old.

Mohini Giriji is a living example of this – having dedicated her life, with love, to the service of thousands of women of all castes and creeds – the poor, the widowed, and the marginalised, across the length and breadth of the country. Her dynamism grows with the years. She is an icon – an ideal woman with a vision, courage and determination, with whom I have worked for many causes over many years. In the Guild, in the AIWC, in the Women's Commission and in the War Widows Association, all of which she headed, she has provided leadership and fought to protect and defend the ideals she stands for. May God bless and keep her for many many more years is my fervent prayer.

The Guild of Service – her brainchild, celebrates its Golden Jubilee this year, with a glorious record of service, providing love, care, and shelter to those neglected and rejected by our cruel society. I congratulate her and her dedicated team that has made it what it is today – a beacon of light and hope to countless women. May the Guild grow as it moves towards its centenary.

15
A Perspective in the Evening of My Life
Margaret Alva

Ageing is a natural process which every human faces. Individuals, families, societies, and governments have to respond to the challenges it poses. Longevity in India in general is on the rise. But the fact that women are outliving men has led to what can be termed as the "Feminisation of Ageing." Compared to elderly men, more than double elderly women live alone, with the poor, aged, single woman suffering the most.

The fear of the pandemic has compelled us to stay home. The streets are largely deserted, meetings avoided, and social contact limited, making us feel lonely and helpless. And I sit back in the quiet luxury of my home – alone. There are times when I ask, "What am I living for?". The memories of the past come crowding in – childhood, school, growing up years, marriage, children, career, work, battles fought, successes and defeats, achievements, and retirement – I have gone through it all.

I came into politics in 1969 at the age of 27 – a young wife, mother, and daughter-in-law, in the shadow of my mother-in-law Violet Alva's sudden and tragic passing away. They were challenging times. The Congress Party had split, Indira Gandhi expelled, and a new left of the centre agenda presented with the "Garibi hatao" slogan, that electrified the nation. The people, young and old, urban and rural, men and women – rallied to create a new India under the leadership of Indira Gandhi. I became part of it.

Over the next 50 years I became a vocal political activist, came to Parliament, worked in the Party, and became a known face in the women's movement. I made my contributions whether in government or outside, championing the cause of women's development and social justice. With Mohini Giri, Padma Seth and Aruna Asaf Ali among others as partners and mentors, we launched campaigns like the Anti Sati Movement in Rajasthan, the initiative for the protection of the girl child in SAARC, amendments to laws affecting women and children and the historic Constitutional amendments for Panchayati Raj and the Reservations for women. They were exciting days. We saw women all over the country emerge from centuries of seclusion and take centre stage.

I worked under four Prime Ministers – Indira Gandhi, Rajiv Gandhi, P. V. Narasimha Rao and Manmohan Singh, in various capacities… and under six Congress Presidents holding posts from the block to the national level. My life changed dramatically when I was appointed Governor of Uttarakand, later shifting to Rajasthan. I had to follow rules of protocol and be cautious in what I said and did. But I refused to be confined. I went out, met people inside and outside the Raj Bhavans I occupied. In fact, I held charge of 3 states at one time – Rajasthan, Goa and Gujarat, a record of sorts.

I returned to Bangalore on my retirement in 2014. I have kept myself occupied with many activities both private and public, though devoting a major part of my time to care for my husband whose health was slowly but surely declining, until he passed away in 2018. He was my strength and support who always stood by me, advising, and encouraging me through the ups and downs I faced. With him gone, I feel lost and helpless.

But during those years, I completed my autobiography *Courage and Commitment* which was released on 19th July 2016 at Bangalore in a memorable event that brought together friends, family, and former colleagues. The book has been well received for its honest account of my life and times.

Friends, relatives, and colleagues tell me, there is so much more I can and must do. Yes, I can and perhaps, I should. I am an outgoing person by nature, happy with people around me. I have lived life on my own terms, to the full, traversing from a small town to reach Lutyens' Delhi, Parliament and Raj Bhavans. I have mentored and helped many to move up. I have been around the country and the world. At meetings and conferences, I have made my contributions and called for a new world order of justice and peace. I have spent over half a century in the Congress Party, 30 years of it in Parliament both in government and opposition.

All through those 50 years, I dreamed of and worked for a new India, where freedom, amity and unity would prevail, and the Constitution and the Law Courts would guarantee and protect my fundamental rights and freedoms. We amended laws, passed new ones, mobilised marginalised groups. We amended the Constitution from time to time to incorporate the aspirations of the new generation, created institutions, built infrastructure, debated issues in our Assemblies and Parliament, created grass roots leadership, brought hope to women, minorities, the Dalits and the tribals, fought for their rights, and brought in new progressive policies. We were proud of our heritage. Where have they all gone? Can I bring them back? We are told nothing existed before 2014!!

What do I see today? The silent majority accepting all the injustice, communal violence, rape and dishonor of women, the hunger and misery of the poor and marginalised and the destruction of the idea of a Secular State. It is slogans, promises, and a mindset hostile to a differing point of view. Criticism is termed anti-national, protests as sedition. Universities are shut, people's movements suppressed, women raped, killed, and made invisible. National assets are sold, banks are looted, the favoured few plunder, and then run abroad, while those in the charmed circle garner every conceivable source of money making.

Our history books are recast to present a particular ideology. Memories of the heroes of the freedom struggle wiped out and replaced by those the government thinks fit. Even the national capital is to be rebuilt, like a mad monarch attempted in our not-too-distant past. There is no discussion or debate. It is a "one party, one man rule".

There is fear; there are threats; there is a sense of hopelessness. My dreams lie shattered, my motherland bleeds, my fellow citizens weep. If you speak, you are a "Deshdrohi" and sent to jail. What are we headed for? Can we expect this reign of terror to end in our lifetime?

It is the young, the new generation, that must now rise - like our freedom fighters did - and be prepared to pay the price. They fought foreign forces that kept us in chains. We have now to fight internal forces that seek to put us back in chains. Religion is not the answer to our poverty, unemployment, violence, hatred, and exploitation. We need to come out boldly, speak up loudly, and die if we must, to ensure the unity and security of our people. This is my prayer, this is my dream.

To quote Tagore:

Where the mind is without fear
and the head is held high,
where knowledge is free.
Where the world has not been broken up into fragments by narrow domestic walls.
Where words come out from the depth of truth…..
Where the mind is led forward by thee
into ever widening thought and action.
Into that heaven of freedom, my father,
LET MY COUNTRY AWAKE!"

Freedom is my birthright and no one can take it away from me.

16
Ageing Gracefully
Major General (Retd.) Ian Cardozo, AVSM SM

"And at the end of it all,
it is not the years in your life that matter,
it is the life in those years."

– Abraham Lincoln

Ageing gracefully is an art. To some it comes naturally, to others like me it took time to acquire. Concepts of 'how one ages gracefully' may differ from person to person – specially an army officer like me, who had to face challenges not common to the average citizen.

The day I retired from the army I decided that I would begin life afresh. In the armed forces we retire when we are quite young. I retired as a Major General at the age of 56. At that age, my civilian counterparts were not even close to the peak of their careers. I felt I had been superseded for promotion for the wrong reasons and that I needed to prove to the world that I was as good, if not better than those who had superseded me. I had done that in the past when I had got disabled in war, so why could I not do that again?

After a while however, I asked myself what did I want to do with what remained of my life? Did I want to impress others that I was better than them? Would that not mean that I would get into the same, mad, rat race of competing with others? Would winning once again give me the satisfaction I was looking for? Ultimately however, that was the way it happened. Proving to myself and the world that I was not redundant became my priority. Prior to retirement, I had sat down one day and opened a file on what I thought I would do on retirement. I pulled out that file and looked at it. On it, in big block letters was written 'Plans for Retirement'. The file included a bucket list of all the places in India and the world that I wanted to see and all the things I had wanted to do but could never do.

As a way of life, nothing could come close to life in the Army. However, it had its limitations. Out of my 35 years service in uniform, 18 had been spent in operational areas and at one time the family was located at five different places. Money was never enough, and I had to take loans from my provident fund to pay for the children's education and the Delhi Development Authority constructed flat that I had acquired, and the loan instalments were still being paid after I had retired.

During my time in the Army, I had taken part in three wars, and I had lost a leg in the Indo-Pak war of 1971. During recuperation at the Artificial Limb Centre at Pune, we were told that we could not return to our units due to our being disabled. We were encouraged to get invalided out of the Army and take advantage of the various concessions offered by the central and state governments. If we chose to stay, then we would serve only at desk jobs and promotions were minimal. Only two officers had been promoted on the staff since World War II and that was abysmal. I felt that the policy that dealt with battle casualties was grossly unfair. We were being denied the opportunity to prove that although physically disabled, we were no less than the non-disabled. I needed to prove to army headquarters and the world that although we battle casualties and were physically disabled, our souls, minds and hearts were invincible and we could prove our ability, provided we were given a chance. What irked me was that those of us, who were part of the victorious army that had liberated East Pakistan, were now left out and in the process of being consigned to oblivion. We felt that the Army was conveying to us that it didn't need us anymore because we were disabled. That hurt and we felt demeaned.

Some battle casualties accepted the option to leave the army in order to access what the central and state governments were offering. These included allotment of land, educational concessions for children, gas agencies and petrol pumps to a lucky few, and jobs for those who were educationally qualified. However, that meant that we had to accept being invalided out of the Army and that did not appeal to me. I had joined a great regiment – the 5th Gorkha Rifles and had fought three wars. No one who has never undergone the experience of war and leading men into battle can ever understand the closeness and camaraderie that evolves with companions with whom one has faced death repeatedly in battle. Our lives thrived on this closeness, and we were now being told that we could not go back to them and that command of troops was denied to the war-disabled. I resented this and decided to challenge the system and prove that the war-disabled were as good if not better than the non-disabled; but at that time I did not know how I would do this.

While I was in hospital recovering from my wounds, a Red Cross sister had lent me a book from her library about the life of Douglas Bader, a Royal Air Force pilot. The title of the book was *Reach for the Sky*. Bader had lost both his legs in an accident but went on to fly Spitfires in World War II. He became an 'Air Ace' by shooting down 23 German aircraft. If he could do that minus both legs, then why could I, who had lost only one leg, not do something similar in my role as an infantry officer? Life moved on. My course mates were promoted to Lieutenant Colonel's rank. Although I had passed out high in my course, I remained a Major and was superseded by those very much junior to me because the policy for war wounded officers had not yet evolved. I felt that I was being punished for being wounded in war. Finally, I was promoted to Lieutenant Colonel's rank but on the staff, more than two years after all my course mates.

In the meanwhile, I had decided that I would adopt a two track strategy. One, to get back to the command of troops by proving that I was physically capable and secondly, if that did not work, then I would get educationally qualified before leaving the service to get a job in the corporate sector. At that time, the qualification on passing out from the National Defence Academy was Inter-Arts/Science which was neither here nor there. So, I went back to school and in the next few years, I managed to acquire a degree in Commerce, a diploma in Personnel Management, an MBA and an MSc in Military Science. Those years were tough. I used to scooter down to Delhi University in Old Delhi after office hours and reach home late at night. Fortunately, I had the support of my wife despite the fact that I could hardly spend time with her or the children during those years. Willy-nilly, I was not only competing with myself to raise my level of academic competence but I was also competing with others to prove that persons with disability were as good if not better than the non-disabled.

One day, while serving at army headquarters, a circular was issued requiring all officers to do the physical proficiency test. Being in low medical category, I did not have to do the test, but I needed to prove to myself and to others that I was no less than the others in physical fitness. I did well in the test and better than seven others in the 2 mile run. Two years later during a tenure in military operations, I had to accompany the Vice Chief of Army Staff on a tour of Jammu & Kashmir. While there, I climbed to a post which was at a height of approximately 4,000 feet. The Vice Chief who landed at that post in a helicopter was impressed and he spoke to the Army Chief stating that I could walk, climb and run and that therefore there was no reason why I could not command a battalion. The Chief directed that I should accompany him on a tour to Ladakh. There, I clambered over snow and ice. On our return to Delhi, the Chief asked for my file and directed that I and all war-disabled officers be given command of units provided they were not taking shelter from their wounds. I was lucky that the Army Chief based his decision on hard facts and that he was not the type to run to the bureaucracy – army or civil - to take such a momentous decision.

By the time I was promoted in command of my battalion, seven years had passed, and I was probably the oldest commanding officer in the Indian army. I had however kept myself fit by swimming and running 5 to 6 kilometres every day. On the first day in command of the battalion, I marched 40 kilometres in the desert. Subsequently I marched 150 kilometres from Kanya Kumari to Thiruvananthapuram. Finally, I rescued a boy from drowning at the beach at Kovalam when no one else felt they had the ability to save him; proving beyond doubt that, in some respects, I was better than the others.

Promotion to Brigadier's rank also proved to be a problem. The military secretary stated that I could not command a brigade as the policy did not allow for it and that there was no precedent. I once again represented to the Army Chief that higher standards of physical fitness were required in lower ranks and if I could command an infantry battalion in peace and on the border then what was the logic in stating that I could not command a brigade? Once again, the Army Chief saw the logic of the situation and gave orders that there should be no restrictions on the promotion of battle casualties and the policy was changed to allow promotion of battle casualties to every rank of the Indian army. It gave me great satisfaction to know that it was I who was responsible for changing the mindset at Army Headquarters in respect of battle casualties and I was subsequently promoted to command an Infantry Division and that too in an operational area. Subsequently, three war disabled officers were promoted to Army Commander's appointments and one of them had lost both legs.

I finally retired as a Major General, as Chief of Staff of a Corps in the North East and looked forward to picking up a good job in the corporate sector. I felt I had all the requisites that met their needs – i.e., a degree in Commerce, a post-graduate degree in Management, other educational qualifications and managing large bodies of men in administrative and operational tasks. What more could the corporate sector need? This is what I thought. I applied for jobs with various companies. The CEOs seemed to be impressed with my qualifications and my experience. They were very polite and said they would call me but that call never came.

What I didn't realise at that time, is that there is a time and place for everything. Perhaps God felt that I had done enough to prove to myself and to others that I was equal to the non-disabled and that the time had now come for me to age gracefully. That meant that the greatest happiness comes in making others happy. He led me to the Spastics Society of Northern India to work for disabled children. One look at those children and I knew that I had found my next vocation. In helping others, I helped myself to get the peace, satisfaction and contentment that had eluded me all those years after I had got disabled.

God has been good to me, and I realised that He had further plans for me. When the door to work in the corporate sector was closed to me, God opened another door. The Government of India had perhaps noticed the work I was doing, and I got a call from the Prime Minister's Office to say that the Prime Minister desired that I accept the post of the Chairman of the Rehabilitation Council of India (RCI). The post was equivalent to a Secretary of the Government of India. There was no salary but by now I had realised that money is not everything. After two years, I was asked to head Helpage which carried a salary and other perks, but I decided to continue to work for the RCI and I recommended the name of an officer who had worked with me in the North-East, who got the job.

After working for nine years with the RCI, I finally retired for the second time, and found that I could still contribute to society through my passion to write. God once again intervened, and I was asked by Roli Books to write the story of the Param Vir Chakra. I worked for two years and gave it my best, and the book '*Param Vir – Our Heroes in Battle*', became a best seller, and has been re-printed twelve times. Other offers to write followed and I have written several other books which have been well received. A good hobby is also a good way to find peace and satisfaction in one's later years. In addition to writing books, I have started writing poems on war which satisfies the creative urge in me. I also realised that good health was very important to age gracefully, and I have been regular with yoga and free-standing exercises. My wife has been my strong support in all my endeavours. Since 2010, I and like-minded battle casualties have been taking part in the 'Dream Run' of the Mumbai marathon and my wife, and some other wives of battle casualties, have joined us as symbols of visible support.

A few other battle-casualties and I continue to work for war-disabled soldiers as part of the War Wounded Foundation and this contribution to the welfare of others brings happiness and satisfaction. There must be many other ways to age gracefully but I have found that making others happy is one of them. Faith and belief in the Almighty is also important. We all need to remember that we are never alone, and with God's blessings we can make the world a better place for ourselves and others. Being happy is, in my opinion the best way to age gracefully and the greatest satisfaction comes from making others happy.

17
Adding Life to Years
Dr. Uma Tuli

I have had the privilege of knowing Dr. (Mrs) Mohini Giri since the establishment of the Guild of Service and as the founder of the War Widows Association where she has worked relentlessly for the elderly and widows to ensure a life of dignity for them.

Dr. Giri has passionately pursued her mission for several years in Delhi, Vrindavan, Srinagar, Rajasthan, Uttar Pradesh, and in many other places. Seeing her deep commitment for the cause it is very clear that people like her never grow old. This is well reflected when we see her in office, sitting straight despite her severe back ache and other problems.

For my own vision of creating a world of equality and full participation for persons with disability, I have derived inspiration from always seeing old age as the "Dawn of Life". As I have added years to my life, I have also learnt to add life to my years. In the process what I have realized is that in order to lead a full life, you have to live meaningfully. Even though old age carries with it certain physical limitations, these can be overcome by determination and reinforcing your will to achieve the goals.

Having to undergo quadruple bypass surgery, when I was 72 years old, I could smilingly tell the doctor "Please go ahead. Hit or miss. I have lived a glorious life and it does not matter if I have to go". I heard people say that I will need to slow down, take it easy – in other words to "watch as the world goes by".

This, I was not prepared to do, as I felt there was much to be done at Amar Jyoti Rehabilitation Centres established in Delhi & Gwalior.

To the question, "What keeps you young?", the answer is very simple. The smiles on the faces of the children, with and without disabilities, playing wheelchair basketball or dancing together. An added joy is to see the deaf blind children communicating easily with children without disabilities. This is the best energy booster ever. What also helps in staying young is to have the good fortune of having dreams and seeing them come true.

When my brother met with an accident in 1965 and lost his leg, the reactions of people made me dream of a society where people accept persons with disabilities. This could be achieved only by providing equal opportunities and full participation to persons with disabilities. Having saved my salary of a lecturer since 1965 in a post office account, we established the Amar Jyoti Charitable Trust in 1981 – the International Year for the Disabled announced by the United Nations. The office was on the roof of my residence and the inclusive school of thirty children with and without disability in equal number was under a tree in Rouse Avenue. The aim was to have a holistic approach to make sure that students have all-round development of their personalities. This concept of inclusion was not well received initially but is being replicated now. With a branch in Gwalior, Amar Jyoti is providing inclusive education to over 900 students who receive medical support, pre-vocational skill development training, inclusive sports and cultural activities, capacity building courses and employment opportunity in one campus. Inclusion has proven to be the ultimate winner. Obtaining social acceptance, proper education and having the latest technology made available to them, our students now are second to none. They have earned several national and international awards.

My growing old never put an age limit on my dreams. The strife and struggle, ups and downs, and countless speed bumps are being faced even today with the same spirit of taking every challenge as an opportunity. Yet another ingredient necessary to add life to years is 'hard work' which you enjoy. Otherwise, work can become a drudgery. To me it has always been a pleasure. Introducing Abilympics in India and organising the Sixth International Abilympics at New Delhi in 2003 was a big challenge but the mantra of convergence of resources made it possible.

Dreams, however, though an individual experience, need many other players – young and old – to be realized. I have been lucky to have a remarkable team who all shared my vision and mission of having an inclusive, barrier-free and rights-based society. Even though a lot of my colleagues and friends with whom I have been associated for over 5 decades are in various stages of ageing, what we have in common is that we are young in spirit, curious and willing to learn and adapt to the ways of this "mad, mad world". Thus, we are able to deal with the rather confusing advances in information technology with the help of younger colleagues, children and grandchildren, who help us patiently. Years ago, we held their fingers to steer them across difficult paths, they now guide our fingers across the new world of keyboards.

I always had a desire to be an all-rounder for which I participated in scholastic and co- scholastic activities. Little did I know that playing badminton, table tennis, basketball etc would help me play with our students and grandchildren as well in my old age. Similarly, being a uniformed person as an honorary Lady Battalion Commander of Delhi Home Guards, the spirit of discipline and making others conscious of it is still very much a part of my life. I am sure this spirit will enable me to march again for 18 kilometers in a Republic Day parade just as I did in 1978 as the first woman to lead the Delhi Home Guards Contingent. The thought of retirement has not occurred yet. As William Hazlitt said: "*The only true retirement is that of the heart; the only true leisure is the repose of the passions. To such persons it makes little difference whether they are young or old; and they die as they have lived, with graceful resignation*".

My faith in God, blessings of Shirdi Sai Baba, and conviction to achieve my mission have given me strength to soar on the wings of inclusion.

So what is old age? It is nothing but a frame of mind, an attitude and a belief. You are as old as you want to be. Nothing more, Nothing less.

18
AGEING
MANI SHANKAR AIYAR

When I was an undergraduate at St Stephen's College, I was sent by the Union, along with a fellow-speaker, to participate in an elocution contest at Delhi College (that is today named after Dr. Zakir Husain). It was a competition in extempore speaking, so each of the participants was called to pick a chit from a bowl and given half an hour's time to prepare his or her remarks. My chit read "Lipstick and Old Age". When my turn came to speak, I began by saying that the handwriting was so poor that I could not make out whether the first word was 'Lipstick' or two words "Lips Stick". I said that I had decided that the subject given to me was "Lips Stick and Old Age", which raised a laugh from the students present, and said there was definitely a link between old age and lips sticking because old age set in only when the individual concerned had nothing particular left to say or, even worse, nothing at all to say! I carried away the trophy for the best speaker at the contest.

This long-forgotten memory came to my mind when my much-respected friend, Mohini Giri, asked me to contribute this article to her issue on "Ageing". For, the fact of the matter is that ageing is not a physical process but a mental and emotional process. One can be old at 20 and young at 80, depending on whether one's faculties are lively and aware or have been put to sleep.

Personally, now that I am nearing 80, my initial reaction was to try to postpone the end of my active life by seeking a post in

Parliament or the Party. I did not consider myself too old for such a responsibility nor was I willing to accept the suggestion, that many members of my family and friends were making, that I should reconcile myself to the end of my political life and not hanker after political posts. Initially, on my retirement from the Rajya Sabha in 2016 after 25 years in politics (15 in the Lok Sabha, 6 in the Rajya Sabha and 5 in the wilderness), I pursued the chimera of a resumption of active politics. I resented being asked to close that chapter of my life, especially the argument that there were no prospects anyway of being restored to activate Congress party politics. It was also pointed out that I had had an unusually long active life: 26 years in the Indian Foreign Service and nearly 26 in politics, making more than half a century of frenzied activity, as against the 36 or so granted to most who had led only a civil servant's career. In my mind, I reversed Omar Khayyam's lines:

What boots it to repeat
How time is slipping underneath our feet?
Unborn tomorrow, dead yesterday,
Why fret about them if today be sweet?

I wrestled within myself with the thought that in my case it was yesterday that was "sweet" while tomorrow stretched into a long tunnel of darkness. I wanted yesterday to continue and tomorrow to be postponed indefinitely. But, however much I wanted to return to yesterday, it was insistently borne in upon me that the Congress party leadership wanted to be rid of me and it was, therefore, a mistaken fantasy to imagine that there would be any political rehabilitation.

While this internal conflict continued in my mind without resolution, the pandemic lockdown was imposed. Whereas, for almost everybody else, the lockdown was a disastrous interruption of their normal lives, I found that the enforced isolation almost compelled me to use the lonely, idle hours to take up the long-pending offer of my publishers to write my memoirs. Somewhat hesitantly at first, and then with increasing momentum, I found

I could push away from my mind my bleak present and future by summoning my past life from the deep recesses of my memory to relive my eight decades on this planet, recalling the good moments and bad and raising a laugh in my head when long forgotten incidents and quips came to mind. Nearly six months into the Covid-19 lockdown, my mood is uplifted, and I feel sixty years younger because, over these months, I have been again experiencing, as in virtual reality, all that has happened to me in the past. I wrote to a novelist friend that I was so grateful to Covid-19 for literally giving me back my life that I was wondering whether to dedicate my memoirs to Covid-19! She was utterly horrified and ordered me to do nothing of the kind.

It will take me at least four months, and perhaps many more, to draw my memoirs to a close, but it has already taught me to view with greater equanimity the prospect of the remaining years of my life. At the passing away of one of the most senior of my colleagues in the Indian Foreign Service, Shri AK Damodaran, someone recited the famous poem:

I strove with none
For none was worth my strife.
Nature I loved, and next to Nature, Art.
I warmed both hands before the fire of Life.
It sinks, and I am ready to depart.

I cannot say the same. I strove with many, and my life was built on such strife. Of course, nature I loved, and next to nature, art. But I am not reconciled to the sinking of the fire of my life, for I find the fire of my life being rekindled in me. I am, therefore, not ready to depart.

As I move to my 80th birth anniversary, I feel energized and full of life. My ageing had accelerated in the four years and more that I had taken to accept the challenge of writing my memoirs. Now that I am doing so, and my time is fully employed, I feel like Lazarus rising from the dead. I feel rejuvenated and believe that ageing happens to others, not, Inshallah, to me. I think I have a decade or more to go but, so long as my mind keeps ticking and my spirits are high, I intend to go on living, not ageing. I have found exemplars in at least three of my seniors who are now in their 90s – K Natwar Singh, K S Bajpai and Maharajkrishna Rasgotra. I hope to remain as young and sprightly as they are.

19
WHAT HAS KEPT ME "TICKING" THESE 97 YEARS?
RAJNI KUMAR

Essentially, I think it has been my love of life. I believe that life is the most precious gift that the human race has been given, and it is therefore incumbent upon all of us to live our lives in the best way possible in order to keep our own lives healthy and to help promote the happiness of humanity as a whole. I have been singularly fortunate to have inherited a strong body and an alert mind from my English family and during the seven decades of my life spent in India. I have had ample opportunities to exploit my abilities and talents and give of my best in my chosen profession of education. It has given me immense satisfaction to see so many students who have benefited from the progressive education that Springdales (the school I founded in 1955) provides and the contribution so many Springdalians are making, to build a better world where all peoples live together in harmony and peace. My involvement with the school has helped considerably in helping my mind 'to tick.'

There is no doubt that when 'old age' descends upon you it brings with its certain problems that cause a lot of irritation - for example your legs don't work as well as they did, your memory starts failing, you have to depend on people doing things for you, and for those of us who are fiercely independent and who have always taken pride in that, it becomes quite difficult to accept this change in our lives. The main question is to keep up a positive spirit, to occupy our minds in a fruitful manner and keep our irritations in check.

I am fortunate at the age of 97 to be living with my family members, my daughter and grand-children and now, a little great grand-daughter. This in itself, is a great boon for there is nothing worse in old age than to be alone. Loneliness is not something I suffer from. I have received every support from my family especially from my daughter, Jo, so I have never suffered from any loneliness or neglect. In fact I have received so much love and care, and this also has been a major factor in making my life such a meaningful and joyous experience.

When you live as long as I have, you naturally have to cope with the ageing process It is most important to occupy our minds as much as we can and not to moan and groan about our failing eye-sight, our poor hearing, our wobbly legs. Also to try to be as independent as possible. Fortunately, in this modern age there are so many gadgets that are available to help one along: hearing aids, a stick to walk with, false teeth, glasses. I have had knee replacements on both knees, I have a lens in one eye for short vision and in the other for long vision, so I have no problem in enjoying my favourite occupation - reading! I have a large collection of books, and my daughter and grandchildren are always providing me with books on subjects of my interest. One of them is tennis, and I never miss watching the Grand Slams and other tennis tournaments on T. V, and then reading the biographies and autobiographies of the tennis stars: Serena, Andre Agassi, Federer and Nadal.

My stick helps me to get around on my wobbly knees. I also have a battery of old students in the medical profession who give generously of their medical expertise whenever required. I really don't know how I would cope without them.

But most important is to keep our minds ticking, and there are many ways of keeping them active – e.g., the radio, the television, "Alexa", and if one is fortunate enough, loving family members to converse with, play cards or word games, as well as a garden to walk in. Pets are also great companions, but they need to be looked after well. There is really no better way of refreshing our minds than by enjoying the beauty of flowers and trees and to hear the chirping of birds. What did the poet write? "One is nearer God's heart in a garden than anywhere else on earth." I watch the News and Shows – especially travel shows and tennis matches on television, I read, play Scrabble and chat with my family members and look forward to celebrating my centenary in March 2023. While there's life, there is hope!

To sum up, my advice to my fellow senior citizens is to keep up a positivity of spirit, to remain cheerful in spite of setbacks, and to develop as many interests as possible to keep the mind alert and the body healthy. Remember, our life - the greatest gift given to us - is more in our own hands than in the hands of the Almighty! It is up to us to make it worth living!

So with hope in our hearts let us all go on "ticking", and all work together to help make a better world.

20
I Love My Age
Zakia Zaheer

As I think of old age, I remember an anecdote I heard long back.

An old lady was sitting and reading the newspaper quietly. She looked up and asked her son to explain something she could not understand. The son explained, though she could not understand his explanation. After some time, she asked him again. The son got irritated and replied curtly. This time, she could not understand anything he'd said, so asked him a third time. Now the son got really angry, and said rudely, "Why can't you get it?! How many times should l tell you?!" The mother said nothing but quietly got up and left. She came back after 5 minutes with a diary in her hand with its page opened at an entry of 40 years ago. She quietly handed it to her son. It read, "Today my son asked me a question 12 times and l replied each time patiently."

Everyone grows old. No one can control the passage of time. But one can embrace old age grumbling and moaning, or gracefully. In my life l am lucky that I have enjoyed each phase of my life, childhood, youth, middle and now old age. Old? Who says l am old? 85 is just a number. I feel l am still young, beautiful, and attractive. I love to dress up, to wear matching bangles, to recite romantic poetry, and even to flirt if possible.

Each phase has its own charm. The freedom of childhood, the intoxication of youth and the responsibilities of middle age and motherhood. The secret is to be positive. I enjoy my freedom from responsibilities. I enjoy playing with my grand children without the responsibility of disciplining them. I enjoy the freedom to get up or sleep late. l enjoy writing: poetry, plays, articles, reading poems & even romantic novels, and cuddling with my grandchildren and telling them self invented fairy tales and see their eyes shining with wonder.

So every age has its charm and now l am discovering that old age is the most comfortable, but only if you have a positive attitude.

I know not how many more years of this bliss l have now, as Ghalib said

"*Rau meinhairakesh e Umar jahandekhiyethamay*
Nay hath bag pehai, ne pa hairakabmein

"The fast moving horse of life is galloping away. I know not where it will stop.

I don't have my feet in the stirrups; nor the reins in my hands."

उमर का बड़ना दुस्तूरे जहाँ है.
महसूस ना करें तो बड़ती कहाँ है
उमर को अगर हराना है तो
शौक ज़िंदा राखीए
घुटने चले या ना चलें
मन उड़ता परिंदा रखीए
मुश्किलो का आना तो पार्ट ऑफ लाइफ है
उसमें से हंस कर बहार आना यही आर्ट ऑफ लाइफ है

21

LIFE'S JOURNEY IS ONE OF EVOLUTION

SUSHMA SETH

Throughout our lives we are seeking, learning and experience.

Like sponges, we absorb ideas and teachings of others, whom we admire and appreciate, whose discoveries and values impact us. Gradually we use this information to form opinions of our own. We cultivate our own philosophy of life, which we tend to follow and express!

Age is a measure of time not of health. But the idea of ageing is feared as a slow decline of mental and physical faculties. It is important to disregard these ageing myths, and cultivate an optimistic mindset, and take steps towards healthy action for long term well-being. We need to disregard the outlook that ageing is unavoidable deterioration. This renewed ageing perspective from pessimistic to optimistic requires us to take health-promoting action and diet.

Wishing to be younger is denying ourselves the beauty of life in the present.

Every decade brings with it wisdom, change and growth. Sixty is definitely not an age to retire from job/work !! At that age, there is a storehouse of wisdom and knowledge, based on confronting failures and savouring success. This is the time to channel one's focus on social, local, creative causes.

Physical fitness is lost during long periods of inactivity, particularly due to illness.

Our body has an infinite capacity for change and renewal. One can achieve total transformation by changing harmful energy patterns/lifestyles that are the cause of weakness, ill health and helplessness. By following certain disciplines, we can transcend the obstacles that afflict our body and mind.

Fitness -enhancing stretches and limbering exercises had been part of my daily routine. At the age of 40 I discovered the ultimate healthy life style– the blueprint for life – the Ashtang Yoga by Sage Patanjali.

These eight points were:

Yam: Ethical discipline. Non-violence, truth, non-stealing/ hoarding.

Niyam: Purity of mind and body. Contentment, Performing duties with diligence.

Asana: Physical stretches and postures – which remove restlessness instability, laziness and obesity. The asanas exercise every part of the body including the organs, which is not offered by any other discipline.

(The asanas should be performed initially under the guidance of a competent Yoga instructor. My teacher was Shri Anil Jha-phone number -9811215936. He has a network of able instructors all over Delhi)

Pranayam:Yogic breathing. Filling the lungs with fresh air, it helps in removing coughs and colds, and diseases related to the heart, lungs and the brain. it also strengthens the epiglottis.

Pratyahar: Control of the sense organs. To resist material desires.

Dharna: Concentration on a single point or on a task in hand. The practice of dharana should move from tangible to intangible, from visible to invisible.

Dhyan: meditation. On the Ajana chakra, or an energy centre of the body.

The seven chakras are Sahasrara (crown chakra), Ajana (third eye chakra), Vishudh (throat chakra), Anahat (heart chakra), Manipura (chakra at the solar plexis), Swadishthan (sacral chakra), Mooldhara (Root chakra).

Samadhi: when the individual soul becomes one with the universal soul. Moksha.

Dhyan:(Meditation)

The most auspicious time for meditation is during Bhram Mahurat, which is between 4 am-6 am: this is a period of silence.

Sit in a comfortable straight back chair or couch or floor if possible in Padma asana.

Close your eyes. Place both hands in Gyan mudra –tip of the fore finger lightly touching the tip of the thumb, keeping the other three fingers straight.

In this mudra, the flow of energy is directed towards the astral body. Intellect develops, memory improves and spiritual development is enhanced.

Meditation apps are available on iPhones under 'Silence Finder.'

In order to incorporate this discipline in my daily life, I was required to wake up at 4 a. M. My routine was as follows: 5-6 am Meditation. 6-7.30 Yagasanas and Pranayam. 7.30-8 am brisk walk!

9 am Leave for shooting / rehearsal/ teaching at Convent of Jesus & Mary, where I taught elocution and drama. The entire routine gave me energy and positivity.

There are always moments to laze and reasons not to exercise-temptations to sleep late, I reserve all this indulgence for Sundays!

A gap of an hour is necessary after doing the exercises and breakfast.

I also opted to become a vegetarian. I belong to a Mathur Kayasth family where non-vegetarian recipes and cuisine are of paramount importance! They feature on top of the list in all conversations and celebrations – I was a problem to feed!!

Fasting cures most physical ailments. Fasting with only water and juice, the body goes into a reparatory mode.

Our stomach is the size of our fist and it is elastic, the more we eat the larger it grows. The body does not require too much food unless one is an athlete/ wrestler/weightlifter. Excess food leads to obesity and ill-health – and it is the MOST difficult task to lose weight! I learnt that, when as a student at college in U. S. A. I had indulged my sweet tooth and added kilos and rolls of fat! It took me 3 years to lose that excess weight.

The main meal should be during the day, either breakfast or lunch. The other meals should be light. We should try to resist snacking between meals!

Our eyesight improves with exercises and palming. Sit in an upright chair, facing east, midst foliage and flowers, if possible! The following exercises should be done very slowly and without straining the eyes.

1. Very slowly look up, then down 3 times.
2. Move the eyes to the left and slowly to the right 3 times.
3. Then move the eyes in a circular fashion – clockwise 3 times then anti- clockwise 3 times.
4. Then focus on a distant object, slowly refocus on a nearby object- the right hand can be used to shift focus.

After the eye exercises, rub both the palms together, cup the palms and place on the eyes, for 5 minutes. Ensure that no light is visible on the covered eyes.

Over a period of time – there is a brightness in the eyes and eyesight definitely improves! Do not expect results immediately and impatiently!

In our Vedas, there is a shloka –

"*Ayam me hasto bhagva, nayam me bhagvatarah: Ayam me vishvabheshjo yam Shiva bhimarshan*" – Atharvaveda IV.13.6.

"Felicitous is this, my left hand, yet more felicitous is this, the right one. This hand contains all healing properties, its gentle touch brings peace and welfare.

(In the palms of our hands, we are given the power to heal and soothe. This has been advocated in the far East as Reiki) We can ask for this healing power – to heal ourselves and other's situations, and conditions.

The state of mind and spiritual development have an intimate relationship with physical health. All conative and cognitive organs take their orders from the mind.

The mind draws its life force from the soul.

Some Observations and Suggestions

Energy follows thought. We attract what we think or speak– whether it is positive or negative.

Laughter and happiness is infectious – as is depression. A smile will invite a smile in response.

Forgiveness is easier to endure than burning enmity. Forgiveness brings calm and positivity.

No one can take away our physical pain or emotional grief, we have to endure it.

Repeating it – magnifies it.

To improve memory and prevent dementia –Memorize 2 lines of a poem/prose/ song daily.

Be cautious on slippery surfaces to prevent falls. Avoid haste. Hold bannisters or take support when ascending and descending staircases.

In this pandemic, here is a concoction and immunity booster: boil in two cups of water – Tulsi leaves, turmeric, grated ginger, cinnamon powder, bay leaf, pepper and large cardamom, till it reduces to one cup. Share and drink it hot.

Each individual is unique – their heredity, environment, bio-chemical structure and mental capacity. The basic strength of these suggestions, based on personal

experience, is a broad guideline.

I pray it helps!

22
Learning Shifts and Creativity Stays
Shanno Khurana

I feel even at 90, i have remained as creative and contributing a member of society since 60 as I was when I was younger. I can't do as much as I once did in a day, but I think what I do is more carefully done, and hopefully has as much meaning. I was widowed at 62. I had married my husband even before I was 18. In my early 60s, when I lost my greatest support, love, my companion, I had to think again about how would one survive? Actually, there was an even bigger question: why does one even need to survive? Music has been my constant companion in my long life, and I know my music is ultimately in God's hands. It is my work and my daily practice—and I am very grateful I have been able to continue to be able to work all my life.

I have tried to use it or shape it in such a way that it satisfies me and is also something that proves useful, beneficial to society. The social acceptance and even appreciation has been very encouraging. Who does not like appreciation? It gives us the incentive to improve whatever we are doing. Yet when age catches up it is difficult to carry on with the work in the same way. This becomes even more difficult when you have been in the public eye for decades and your audience expects you to perform in the same way as you once did. And it would have become absolutely impossible for me to carry on if I had to suffer irrelevance, or complete public rejection. At the same time, it would also have been completely impossible for me to carry on if I expected the same level of public attention for my work as I did when I was younger.

Ageing can be difficult for someone in the public eye, one who is expected to perform a certain character or have a certain presence or persona, because ageing will demand a shift in that image, and the media and public may not take to that shift, leaving you without the professional appreciation which is necessary to carry on working. One has to learn how to shift one's image and continue to serve in a new way that is both honest to one's own needs as well as useful and meaningful to the people or the public whom you are serving. During my 60s and 70s I still managed to travel widely and give concerts in Europe and the United States which were perhaps some of the most classically rigorous and meaningful recitals I have given in my career. Importantly the wisdom to communicate the depth of one's music only really sets in later in one's career. However by the time I was in my 80s travelling became harder. I also gradually changed my repertoire. And most importantly I am not sorry at all for making these shifts or changes in myself and my music.

I find the acceptance of my relatives and dearest friends gives me strength. No matter how difficult the challenges, they have helped tide me over the times when my body and mind do not cooperate, and watched me as I try to find new ways to satisfy myself. After all, what has to happen will happen. This is easier said than done but the sooner you realise this, the easier it becomes. This also allows you to adapt to the challenges that come in life and no one who wants to carry on working and contributing can expect not to face challenges. As time moved on I could not even sit cross-legged or squat on the floor to be able to sing. And that was when my daughter Payal who used to design folding furniture made me two stools specially of the height I required — one for me to sit on and the other for me to keep my *tanpura* on. The two stools folded into a suitcase and I was able to ask Rikhi Ram to make me a special *tanpura* that could be folded into another suitcase, and, at the age of 80, I was able to tour the USA giving concerts all across the East Coast thanks to them. Of course, I had support: my disciple Maitreyi, faithful members of my orchestra, and above all, the emotional support I have received from my grandson Naman in all the years ever since my husband died has given me a true second innings in professional life. I just cannot state enough that but for THAT support of my near and dear ones, I could never have managed, it has given me a capacity to endure and accept the changes that were inevitable.

Acceptance of a Changing Self

Apart from the exploration of each raga that I was fortunate to learn from my gurus, one of the most creative aspects of my career from my late 30s through my 50s was the opportunity to compose music for operas. I drew on whatever I was learning in classical music as well as folk music. However in my 60s and 70s, I found myself exploring a different kind of creativity. Perhaps these were of a slightly more learned nature, reflecting on how the aesthetics of music affect the body and mind, and how it impacts art too.

I think it was in 2003, Dr. Kalyan Bagchi, brought out a book, *Music, Mind and Mental Health* that was published by the Society for Gerontological Research with Helpage India. He offered me an opportunity to do some research and experiment, by singing different ragas in different tempos to people of different age groups, to assess what effect music has on them. Some realities of old age were exposed in my research, for which I selected ten categories.* We made charts for the listeners to respond to the impact of words in music to determine whether they were moved by the music or the poetry; and then we had others to assess response to the *abhinaya*, or expressive quality of the music. The role of melody (capturing the '*sur*' aspect) had to be differentiated from what the effect of tempo was. Did the transition from slower to fast tempo

* Khurana, Shanno.)Impact of Music on Body and Mind: a Live Experiment with Special Emphasis on the Elderly, in Kalyan Bagchi (ed.) Music, Mind and Mental Health, Society for Gerontological Research, R-18 Hauz Khas Enclave, New Delhi 16, 2003, pp. 55-66.

alter the mood? This brought us to working only with rhythm, to study the effect of taal. Did something as simple as the elevation of the volume play a part and did the music allow for some kind of visualization? Finally, a question equally needed to be posed whether silence had an effect, and was there a difference to the responses between those above and below 65? In some ways, this was a very gratifying experiment because I, at my age then- which was around eighty- was able to calculate the alertness of my mind as much as my audience's. It was heartening to really know and have the confidence to know that one can change how one sings, or what one sings, and still have a meaningful response from a listener; it gave one confidence to persist and not to give up.

Naman drew my attention towards *Ragamala* miniatures sometime in my late 60s. With him I started looking at the *shlokas* written on top of historical paintings and we found that disappointingly, the words need not have anything to do with the rasa, or mood or the *swaroopof* that raga. Yet, the painting itself captured something of that essence. I remember at a joint lecture-demonstration we did at SOAS in London University in 1997, he showed slides of specific paintings and with each painting I sang compositions in that *raga* that I had learnt that could express that *rasa*. Every raga can be communicated in so many ways and while in my younger days I was interested in exploring those many ways, now, while looking at the mood in the painting, I was able to see which ways were thought to be more suitable. Discovering that the *rasa* could match the paintings very precisely at times was thrilling as it reinforced one's learning and experience through another new discipline. Not only that, we carried our collaboration forward when he curated exhibition on "The Body in Indian Art & Thought" in Brussels in 2013, where he created a special enclosure to show how music and art can be appreciated together. Every time a visitor went in front of a painting music of that raga, like Devgandhar, Deshkar, Bilawal and many others (even the all too rare Deepak) would play for them, corresponding with the painting they were looking at. It was a novel experience.

Musically, I can see that there was a shift. For one, I gradually slipped more into the '*dhyan*' of ragas and not the showmanship to please audiences. My voice became deeper and I had to try and listen to myself to see if the same ideas sounded as pleasing in a lower pitch. This was not always easy and I tried to keep a balance. I found in my 70sand 80s, I became calmer, and I found, unknowingly, my voice and creativeness assumed a greater confidence in what we call '*pukar*' in Hindustani music: opening the voice with abandon at phrases which I now felt expressed the emotive seed or kernel of that raga. At last my audience was 'one' with me and that is when I found '*ananda*' – bliss! It was wonderful to go through this experience, and I loved it as I was now singing with greater abandon.

In government jobs, or corporate ones, a person retires at 60 but I, as a musician in my 70s, 80s- and now even in my 90s- have found myself still exploring new aspects of my creativity. So as a musician one never retired. I am still ticking!!

Apart from love, it is creativity that also gives one energy and strength. If God has granted me long life, I thank him for preserving that beautiful ability to be creative in every sphere of my life, not just in my profession. This nurturing of creativity, protecting its place in one's life, is a constant process and if you protect it, it also protects you. Even today at the age of 93 I find my mind keeps ticking. When I am unwell and bedridden I still keep repeating *sargams* and the *swaroop* of *ragas*, it keeps me company, it keeps me focused and also less forgetful.

It is amazing how with age one becomes forgetful! No matter how many almonds you keep eating early in the morning! I personally feel one has to be brave, mentally, to face the transition from young age to old age. People accept it gradually, these are the realities of life, as we all transit from the realm of young to old. I have no regrets. My music *sadhana* has given me all that I craved for: recognition, fame, love and affection. What else do I want? I suppose there are certain small regrets which will always remain but what has to happen will happen and you cannot do anything about that. This acceptance allows one to also cross those regrets. Yet, I have observed, that whenever I felt I have reached the goal I craved for, the goal actually goes further up, more distant, and I realise I have not reached it at all. To be honest I've never really enjoyed listening to recordings or albums of my music – I can see what I did not do, or what I could have done differently, and by the time I listen to that piece—often I have come up with better note combinations and seen a different aspect to the *raga* which I did not record at the studio. So there is something further to carry on trying for. Is this creating a situation where I am bound to have regrets? I do not know. And then I tell myself: do not be so ambitious; find your peace within; enough is enough; God has given you so much; be thankful to Him!" This is a constant process of negotiation.

Challenges of Old, Equip One for New Ones

There has been no dearth of challenges in my life ever since I entered the classical music world. Not belonging to a musician's family, but to professional service people, consisting of engineers, doctors, lawyers, or those in public service whether in the defence- or foreign services, I found I was not taken seriously as a professional musician in the community of musicians, or even found that my professional needs ran the risk of not being taken seriously amongst my social circle. This was a challenge that I learnt to face relatively early in my career, but it is surprising that it continues to stay as troublesome today as it was 75 years back. Only now, one is more practiced at spotting the prejudiced mindsets.

I found that in spite of my having learnt my music at the feet of great gurus, like Mushtaq Hussain Khan of Rampur Gharana, the eminent musicologist Thakur Jaideva Singh, Dr. S. N. Ratanakar of who was the Vice- chancellor of Indira Gandhi Vishvavidyala at Khairagarh (and one of the most erudite and learned men on the structure of rare ragas), and from Prof. R. N. Musalgaonkar who upheld the rigorous training of the Gwalior gharana, I forever sensed that there was some sort of grudge against me. Sometimes word would get back to me, "Why does the wife of a well known and well to do doctor need to occupy a seat which belongs to us?" The male musicians of my generation only knew of women performers who were *tawaifs*, and that was certainly not the way they could speak to me. Nor were those in senior professional spaces capable of understanding the requirements for hiring or commissioning women. My ways of asking for professional engagements, whether programmes or record-deals, were certainly not the ones that the men in positions of power were used to, nor the methods I was going to employ.

Little did that generation know what kind of struggle lay before a middle-class woman who wanted to make music a profession in India, that behind those well-ironed *khadi* saris was someone who belonged to a family that started from scratch after the Partition of India;a family that was both anglicised and yet intensely proud of its Indian heritage; that behind the very same Shanno Khurana on the concert stage or All India Radio studio was also a kitchen she was cooking for her extended family in, and maintaining her daily *rayaz* even when she had her baby of a few months in her lap and *tanpura* in her hand. Every little paycheque of 25 rupees for a broadcast from Radio and that monthly salary of 75 rupees from Sangeet Bharti for teaching music was making a difference to help support the family. There was that passion, there was my husband's unwavering support, and I guess, yes, there was also the energy of youth, which drove me deeper and deeper into this great music of ours. Probably the many men who ran the industry in those days just did not realize, or could not bring themselves to see, that, behind that passion that drove Shanno Khurana professionally, she also observed her duties as a wife – as Mrs. Khurana – not as Shanno Khurana the professional. We drew our own *lakshman-rekha*: If I wore a sleeveless blouse and a chiffon *sari* to go out to cocktails with her husband, I was equally careful to dress in traditional *saris*, when I performed on stage. And there, sitting in the audience, was my husband, who would stand back after the performances, never introducing himself as the famous Dr. P L Khurana, but always as Shanno Khurana's husband. We were there to help each other through the challenges we faced.

Speaking of being dressed for an occasion — I must mention here a remark made by a lady who was a paid professional music critic for a leading national newspaper, "We used to scrutinise you, we paid attention to what you were wearing, how nice you looked..." I was horrified. Here was a professional, a woman at that, who was paying attention to everything else except the content of my music. The problem of being conditioned to see women in one way was not just stemming from men in our profession but women themselves. Another critic sent by a newspaper once remarked saying, "You looked so nice singing with your sitar!" Not *tanpura*, mind you, she did not know the difference, but had been appointed as a music-critic! It was frustrating. Neither were women being taken seriously, and neither was the profession itself. They say that "f it doesn't kill you, it makes you stronger". Well, perhaps the nature of the challenges we learnt to overcome have given these bones some strength to be able to endure.

Friends, Peers and Colleagues Live On

During the period from the 1950s to the 1970s, I was concerned with bringing the richness of our musical tradition to new audiences through operas and other theatrical or film experiments. In the 1980s, however, I grew more concerned with the condition of female musicians, not just of my generation, but I was seeing that those of my children's age, were still facing the same pressures I had at their age. This convinced me to hold music festivals of, and by, only women musicians—where not just the main musician but even their supporting accompanists were all women. This showed the public that they were as good as men, but it was important to give the musicians themselves the confidence they needed to emerge as professionals. We struggled to raise funds, because unless they were properly remunerated, there would be no point.

However as I grew older, and my music more inward, I began to realise that there were also other concerns I had for the profession as a whole. One of them was that there were many ragas that I myself was hardly getting the opportunity to sing or even hear anymore. These were ragas I had learnt from great masters, and I shifted my repertoire to focus on them in my recitals. This allowed me to reach newer audiences of connoisseurs, and that was a pleasure. Jaldhar Kedar, Malhua Kedar, rare varieties of Malhars, and so many Bhairavs, Sarangs, Bilawalsand Todisand so many others ragas too started featuring in my programmes. By this stage, with growing respect in the profession, I was able to convince the Sangeet Natak Akademi and other professional bodies to start holding festivals of such rare ragas. I realised that like me, other musicians too were not getting to explore these ragas, which ran the risk of disappearing from our repertoire. Our university curricula did not allow students to really learn these ragas and in the culture of instant gratification, our own disciples were not really understanding these ragas either. Again, I am gratified to see that the subject has been taken seriously and now greater attention is being paid to this subject in universities and on the concert stage.

As much as one's music is an inward journey, communicating it is dependent on the collaboration of a team – a dialogue with one's peers. I suppose in the younger days one is so enamoured of the gurus and follows them, but as time goes on one also learns to celebrate what others in our profession have done. I was always very close to Ali Akbar Khan Saheb who was like an elder brother and I tied him a *rakhi* for many decades. Pandit Chaturlal who was my tabla accompanist and Pandit Inderlal as well as Ustad Shakoor Khanon the sarangi accompanists strengthened so many of my ideas through our weekly sessions of *rayaz*, whether or not there was a recital to prepare for. With age, one loses one's friends and peers, and younger musicians learnt to work with me, but I think an extraordinary strength has come from working for decades together with those musicians when one was younger.

I can never forget a performance I gave in Chennai for the Prakriti Foundation about ten years ago. I took on a new challenge, a piece of music called *Taal Sagar* or *An ocean of talas* composed by Pandit Ram Ashray Jha. Panditji and I were the same age, but he died some years earlier. I admired his knowledge and I decided to try and sing his composition. This consisted of eleven *ragas*, where each *raga's* poetry merged, both with its words and *swaroop* into the next and, most importantly, without a break, into a new *tala*, or beat-cycle. The trick was to do it seamlessly without the audience realising that you'd actually slipped into a new beat. I think he would have liked the fact that I tried this on the Madras audience. Carnatic music audiences love keeping rhythm publicly, and they found themselves having to keep constantly shift their counting! The composition started from 16 beats and kept changing 15, 14, 13, 12, 11, 10, 9, 8, 7, and 6. I can never forget that evening. It came from a confidence in knowing those ragas, learning how to sing many *raga-sagars* from my guru Mushtaq Hussain Khan, and the years of experiments with *talas* with Chaturlal and my fellow orchestra members that allowed me, to pull off an experimental piece so much later in life.

Age and experience open new possibilities. I think a maturity of thinking brought a shift in my style of presentation as well as new opportunities. When Zakia Zaheer asked me to set her poem *Main aurat hoon* to music a few years ago, I decided to make it into a little operetta that was quite expressionistic. I got the opportunity to use silence in the music: something I had never really had the opportunity to do before. The silence was a way to 'give voice' in the middle of the music to the atrocities inflicted upon women. And on the other hand, when the music and dance critic, Leela Venkataraman asked me to compose the music for a ballet called *Ganeshaya-Namah*, I knew I would have to play with rhythms that bodies would enjoy dancing to.

Age has not deterred me so far. I remain grateful to God for his blessings, and pray that whenever He comes to take me, I can go on singing.

23

AGEING: THE INDIAN PERSPECTIVE

DR. SYEDA HAMEED

With seven decades of my life having rolled by, these lines of Jalaluddin Rumi, Sufi, mystic poet, haunt me as I step into old age.

Why does a date palm lose its leaves in Autumn?
Why does a full head of hair get bald?
Why is the tall straight figure
Which divided the ranks like a spear
Now bent almost double?
The wrestler who could hold anyone down
Is led out with two people supporting him
Their shoulders under his arms?
God answers
'They put on borrowed robes
And pretend they were theirs
I take the beautiful robes back
So that you will learn the robe
Of appearance is only a loan
Your lamp was lit by another lamp
All God wants is your gratitude for that

This poem by Rumi reflects on ageing, impermanence of the body and transience of our lives. Rumi lived in the 13th century but his poems and his mystic philosophy have lived for centuries, illuminating the universal experience of loss and decay and the ephemerality of life. Like mystics in many religious traditions

Rumi finds meaning in the routine experience of ageing. His images detail the movement from vitality to decline found in every aspect of life. For Rumi the decline into old age is the lesson about who we really are. Ageing is a reminder that the lamp of our existence is actually lit from another lamp. For those who work and live with elders Rumi's message is both practical and relevant.

I was all of 24 years when I began working in the geriatric ward of a hospital in Canada. It was a French Canadian missionary hospital. Christian values of mercy and charity were assiduously practised by the nuns who ran the place. In the wards I was shocked to see old and lonely people longing for company, for a kind word, for a smiling face. That was back in the late sixties when we in India still valued our *buzurgo*. (our elders) I could not understand why my Canadian patients' families were not there to take them home when they were discharged. It was our duty to book a taxi, pre-pay the driver, and ensure a caregiver who would open the door and leave them food at least for the first day.

One saw them everywhere on the streets of Ottawa. In the forenoon they were seen walking slowly on the sidewalks pushing their little carts to the nearest grocery store to buy small provisions, whatever their meagre pensions would allow. Young people walked past them impatiently, intent on their own missions. I looked at this promenade of elders with sadness recalling lines from my favourite poet T. S. Eliot. The poem was called *Love Song of J Alfred Prufrock* about an old man reminiscing about his life. The lines which haunted me then and haunt me today, I want to share:

I grow old I grow old
I shall wear the bottom of my trousers rolled
Shall I part my hair behind, shall I eat a peach?
Shall I wear white flannel trousers and walk upon the beach?

I prayed and prayed, "May I never live long enough to reach the age when I become Prufrock!"

To provide a snapshot of ageing in India, let us begin with some numbers. The population of the senior citizens in 2026 is projected at 173 million according to the office of RGI recorded in Lok Sabha, 2015. According to census 2011 the population of senior citizens was 104 million out of which 53 million were female and 51 million male. In comparison, in 2001 of a total 76.6 million, males were 37.8 million and females 38.9. Going back to the 1961 census the percentage of the senior citizens was 5.6%. In 2011 it increased to 8.6%. According to the 2011 Census, 71% lived in rural areas while 29% lived in urban areas. Their literacy rate was 44% of which 59% were males and 28% females. In rural areas 66% males and 28% of females were working. In urban areas 46% males and 11% females were working. The main diseases of senior citizens were locomotor disability and visual disability. Kerala showed the highest percentage of senior citizens at 12.6 % (2011) and Arunachal and Nagaland the least percentage of senior citizens at 4.6 and 5.2 respectively. NSSO 2004-2005 showed 18 million senior citizens lived below the poverty line. Three decades ago on 14th December 1990 the United Nations General assembly announced that 1st of October will be observed as the International Day of Older Persons. The theme for the 2020 International Day Of Older persons was "Pandemics: Do they Change how we address Age and Ageing?".

When I was part of the Planning Commission of India working on the 11th and 12th Five Year Plan, we recognised the immense potential and wisdom of the elderly and understood the value of their involvement especially in the education of their community. Our directive to Government of India's line departments was to formulate schemes whereby elders could participate in them, such as ECS (Early Childhood Education) for children of their communities. Visiting children in schools to impart to them their knowledge of local history, folk stories, songs, poetry and share with them their wide range of experiences.

The ground reality of the elderly which I saw during my tenure was very stark. A few examples are illustrative. In the

Koraput district of Orissa I saw a line-up of old women at the District Commissioner's office. Upon enquiring I discovered they all were widows who had been rejected by their families. The reason they appeared before the apathetic Babus was to find out if there was an 'empty spot' so they could become eligible for a paltry pension of a few hundred rupees. Thus they were waiting for death. The 'empty spot' was created when a widow died and her pension could go to the next in line. In Pochampally district of Andhra Pradesh (now Telangana) where I had gone to look at the most unique handloom industry, I found an elderly couple sitting on the roadside. That moment would haunt me for months. The woman had lost one eye due to a spindle the other to cataract. All the men possessed were two utensils, one for water one for food, blank faces craving charity of passers. From Chamba in Himachal to Mokokchung in Nagaland, wherever I went, the story was the same.

In the course of our planning we learnt about the 'inverted pyramid' in some parts of the world. In Japan for example, the population of the elderly was increasing while that of the youth was on the decline. So the new media 'game' was 'Adopt a Grandparent'. Elders there have decent social security and pension to tide them over, so they get emotional sustenance by grand parenting, without becoming a burden on the young.

In addition to according them economic and health care rights it is important to address the emotional insecurities of the elderly. The loss of spouse, friends, relatives and overarching loneliness creates a vacuum in life that cannot be shrugged away. In this fast paced, polarised and individualistic world it is essential to create awareness and sensitivity in the young generation towards ageing. Fostering close relationships between the elderly and young is the responsibility of mid generation. It cannot happen on its own; it is a deliberate, calibrated process. Simply saying that there is much that generations mutually learn and imbibe is not enough. This tautology needs to be shed in favour of painstaking effort and showing by example. Youth could be drawn to the wisdom of the elders as much as the elders are to their energy.

The ethos of family 'jointness' was embedded in the assumption that all members in the family have a utilitarian function which assumes that they are beneficial to one another. One ubiquitous example here is in households where elderly take care of children, thereby providing restful spaces to young parents. That concept has also flown away.

Literature, folk and classic, has traditionally been the domain of the elderly; I recall this talent of my *buzurgs* as the best part of my childhood. Listening to grandmothers recite stories from Arabian Nights, Sindbad the Sailor, Mulla Nasruddin, Panchtantra, Gul e Bakawali, Akbar and Birbal, Shaikh Chilli made bedtimes feel like a magic carpet. That culture has yielded space to video games; PUBG and the likes carry crazed kids through wakeful nights. It is time that these giant conglomerates (behind these thrill-bombs) are thrown out of their households by parents, ordinary people across the globe who see their deleterious effects on children. To revive these bygone engagements which are mutually beneficial to three generations is an idea the world needs to focus on.

Alternative medicine has caught global imagination. India, indeed South Asia, was for centuries the repository of this knowledge. Following the sudden interest shown by the West, India also withdrew it from the niche. In the last two decades it was brought into the mainstream after it received global attention. In the market today we hear words like Daadi Ma ke Nuskhey or Nani ka Karha. The culture of home medicines (*jadi booti ka karha*) for cold, cough, constipation etc has emerged out of knowledge which was the domain of elders. Despite this their presence is regarded as burdensome in families which they have nurtured all their lives. Their role in the family is considered unproductive and rarely valued.

Another problem confronting policy makers today is addressing the safety issues of vast numbers of elderly left alone to fend for themselves. Large scale migration from rural to urban, increased nuclearization of families has had a terrible impact on their lives. Metro cities and small towns have seen gruesome cases of violent crimes against the elderly spiralling every day.

The dwindling of the joint family, the rise of dual career families, possible shift in filial piety, increasing life expectancy with greater chances of a prolonged old age characterised by poverty, degeneration, more empty-nest years, and dependency, have all added to the seriousness of the problem. It has made the elderly more susceptible than ever to abusive treatment. Issues of gender and ageing take on a whole new meaning in the patriarchal social system which characterises South Asia. Gender studies have widely documented the subaltern status of older women, victims of violence, discriminated against in all sectors. 90 percent of them are from the unorganised sector which means they have no social safety net, no pension and no provident fund.

It is projected that Asia Pacific will have the world's largest proportion of older persons in the next 30 years. It is thus crucial for us to raise public awareness and formulate and evaluate measures and programs to cope with the demographic challenges. Problems waging across South Asia are similar. The state of their greying populations, juxtaposed with environmental degradation, poverty and food crisis- sweep across this region. SAARC was designed as the Forum where such issues could be raised. Due to confrontational politics between the seven members this Forum has become non-functional.

But instead of half empty, can we see the glass as half full? Could the very elders who sit on 'rejection fringes' be seen as our messiahs for peace? In today's fragmented era, where communities are on a boil, regions targeted, and individuals annihilated for their identity, should we not look at the elderly to help us foster the links of unity and peace? Can they help us bind our societies together? The world is poised on annihilation. Its triggers lie in hands with a proven record of mass destruction. No matter in which part or which political colour, all global citizens want peace. For decades human destruction is planned in boardrooms where men confer with like-minded men, heedless of where their confabulations are leading. Women and elders are always missing. It's time they were folded into the peace process; for the sake of this planet and all its dwellers.

I wanted to conclude with a few lines of poetry to complement age. But wherever I looked there was longing for bygone days of yore. So I moved from literature to life and found what I was looking for. Among my own circle there are a few people who have more life and spirit than those half their age. My role model in many aspects of life, in particular on ageing is a woman called Mohini Girl. She defies all stereotypes and rides the chariot of effervescence and joy. I found the right words for her in lines from Shakespeare's *Antony and Cleopatra*.

Age cannot wither her, nor custom stale
Her infinite variety

Such moulds are uncommon but still 'seek and you shall find'. We need to get our tincture from them as we step happily into old age. Looking to the state to resolve problems of ageing is a solution but the real answer lies within ourselves, within each one individually and collectively.

24
Living in Greater Hope and Positivity
Dr. George Mathew

If I could contribute in a little way in realizing the narrative of ageing, I would be happy to do it by sharing the experiences that I have gained in the 77 years of my life. My focus is on my childhood and the struggle I had to undergo in those days.

I am a person whose thinking and outlook have been shaped by a process similar to making iron and steel; in short, the furnace of life taught me very valuable lessons right from childhood that stood me in good stead. I have passed through immense difficulties, distresses, disappointments, tragedies and hurdles, which, instead of making me desperate, depressed or gloomy, made me more determined to fight life's battles, not only for me and those around me, but also for society as a whole.

A person needs rock-like faith, confidence and motivation to face life's trials. That is where the connection between mind and body comes. My life experience shows that age becomes just a number if one can develop a positive attitude and mind, optimism, the ability to see everything good in others as well as the world, and work accordingly.

Though I lacked most of the comforts in life that can make one's childhood or youth happy, I was blessed by the fact that I received strong motivation from my parents to work hard for others and society. I was their first child born after seven years of marriage. They had to bear much mental pain, stress and strain in those days for many years, and hence they had taken a vow to dedicate their first child to do God's work through the church in the Biblical tradition. Finally, their prayers were answered. But I was born a premature baby in 1943 in a village in Kerala and due to the absence of any worthwhile medical facilities, my mother's family and relatives thought I had little chance of survival. Hence, I was baptized in the church much earlier than the prescribed time. As per the church tradition, if an un-baptized child dies, the body has to be buried in the home land, as the church cemetery is not available. But I survived. I survived through all gloomy predictions, not only then, but all throughout my life's journey of ups and downs.

I inherited many qualities from my parents, who were teachers, especially from my mother who was iron-willed. She was widowed when she was just 39 in 1959. My father died at the age of 44, leaving me, then aged 15, and six of my younger brothers to fend for ourselves. We lived in a rural hill area near the forests (Kumplampoika) in Quilon district, Travancore (Central Kerala today). In 1944, when my parents settled in that village in a hut, we didn't have basic facilities like electricity or water, and even essential items like rice were in short supply. My mother had to go to a distant place by foot to teach in a government primary school while my father taught in a school, about three miles away. But he had to resign his job because of health issues and started a small shop in our village, which ultimately landed us in huge debts and liabilities.

While my father was running the shop, I was studying in the nearby High School. One day he was taken all the way to Trivandrum medical college for treatment. The doctors told my uncle that he would not survive and so he was brought back to our home where he passed away on March 18, 1959. The next day was my Secondary School Leaving Certificate (SSLC) examination. I could not appear for it and lost one year of my studies. Then I appeared for the mid-year examination in September that year and passed SSLC.

With my father's death, my life entered a very difficult phase. I had to wind up the mini-merchandise and prepare for my exams six months away. There were lots of debts to clear off and I made door-to-door visits frequently to collect money from those who had taken goods from my father's shop on loan. I also had to work for meeting the daily needs of my six younger brothers and many other challenges. Anyway, by that time we had a house in place of the old hut. That strong roof over our heads was one of the greatest blessings we had, thanks to the help and support of our extended family. But there was hardly any money left to plan anything even for the next day. We had to live on the meagre salary earned by my mother as teacher in the primary school.

What to do after passing the High School examination was a big question mark before me. Going to a college for studying was expensive. I didn't even have foot wear in my childhood because of lack of money. Some of those whom I consulted about my further studies in our parish and neighbourhood advised me to limit my studies to become a primary school teacher. Training for primary school teachers was available in a village-centre four miles away and thereafter a primary school teacher's job was a possibility in the nearby school. But my dream was to study in one of the best colleges in Kerala.

Of course, my dream was nurtured by my parents who wanted to give me the best education possible. My ideas gained strength, also because I was exposed to the social realities around us with my active involvement in social and religious issues through the parish. My contacts with the best minds of the time in our area were possible from a young age because I was sent to attend boys' camps, meetings and conferences. That way, I received good exposure to the outside world, which otherwise would not have been possible for a person living in such a remote area. I used to take Malayalam books from the 'Bodleian Library' in our village and read them late into the night with the kerosene lamp.

I had heard of young students from well-to-do families in our area studying in colleges in far away towns. They had money which I lacked. But I got support from my relatives to study in a prestigious college – Union Christian (U. C.) College, Alwaye, near Cochin (now Kochi), about 120 km from home. I made the best use of it for one year and became Secretary of the hostel where I stayed and utilized every hour and opportunity to meet people to see and understand new situations and conditions of life. Due to financial difficulties, I studied only for one year in the Union Christian College. Then I got admission in the Catholicate College, Pathanamthitta, some ten kms from our home, to pursue my BA degree course. I was concerned that my six younger brothers also must get college education as they were growing up. As a day scholar, I travelled by bus with a student concession ticket-- 10 paise one way-- for three years while I was in the college. Extracurricular activities in schools and colleges, including elocution competitions, made me busy all the time. All these proved crucial in developing in me some sort of a quest for leadership as well as articulating my ideas and establishing a wide circle of friends.

The three-year college education was a period of hard training and learning in every way, including instilling in me rigorous discipline upholding the time-tested values and principles of life. Money to meet all our educational and daily requirements was a big problem and we had to tighten our belts as the only steady income was our mother's salary and some support from our close relatives. We often toiled in our farm to cultivate agricultural products to keep the wolf from the door. Sometimes, it was even difficult to find ten paise to meet the bus fare and there were times when I walked all the way from the college to our home to save that money. But these limitations did not stop me from my pursuit to achieve something good in life and change the scenario for the better. I knew that there was no short cut to success and the only way was to work hard day and night with commitment and dedication. These ideas were inculcated in me by my parents, extended family, teachers, community, including the parish, and our relations. These were imparted to my six brothers also and they have followed suit.

Lack of money also did not prevent me from fully utilising my limited abilities for leadership along with my studies. I was elected as the College Union Secretary through a party-based students' union election during my final year in the college. I made a mark, winning the confidence of the students, teachers and college authorities. The students' union election is always a difficult task. One of the dignitaries whom I had the honour to bring to the college to address the students was the then Governor of Kerala, His Excellency Shri V. V. Giri. Sharing the stage with the Governor as well as several other dignitaries during my one-year term as the Union Secretary was a great inspiration and confidence-building step for me. I passed out of the college with second class in BA Economics, which was a tough proposition in those days, especially when we had no electricity in our house and had to burn midnight oil with the kerosene lamp.

I was aware of the social mission I was entrusted with from a young age and my mind never wavered from that goal. My thinking and ideas were rooted in the social systems and realities of the times and as I grew up I realised where the fault lines lay in the religious and political spheres and I wanted to change them and correct them in the best way possible. In all my activities, speeches, writings and discussions at various forums and platforms, I formulated and explained my ideas and won recognition and acceptance in social and intellectual circles. While in college I also wrote short stories to highlight my ideas and received prizes as well.

After passing BA, I worked as Secretary of the Students Christian Movement (SCM) of India, based in Trivandrum (now Thiruvananthapuram), for three years. I wanted to help my mother and brothers by improving the home finances, though my salary was meagre. I used to move around the city on a bicycle to meet people and organise meetings and discussions in colleges and the university. I came into contact with youth leaders and eminent people in the city and organised various orientation and cultural programmes for the students and teachers. One memorable event was a musical concert by the famous singer Yesudas which I organised for fund raising. Although some serious problems developed in the conduct of the musical concert, I withstood them. With the money thus mobilised, we bought land for building a students centre. The SCM centre in the capital city of Kerala says it all. In the process, I learnt step-by-step: how to organize programmes or major events, how to speak, how to write and debate. Developing skills, contacts with higher social groups, having a wider vision of the world and awareness of the opportunities lying ahead, were necessary conditions for me to go foreward.

After the three years of my work in the SCM Trivandrum, I realised that to equip myself to fulfil my social mission, I must study more. But I had no financial resources to go for post graduate studies. However, through a long process and contacts, I could join a prestigious theological college in the Bangalore city for the three year Bachelor of Divinity (B. D) course. The liberal theological studies under outstanding International scholars and professors from many countries enabled me to look at religion and society with a difference.

Then my question was how to use religious platforms for social and church reforms. After I got the theological degree, I joined the Ecumenical Christian Centre, Whitefield, as Programme Secretary and conducted several national and international conferences on topics of relevance then. I could bring eminent persons of that time like Jayaprakash Narayan, I. K. Gujral, O. V. Vijayan, Mrinal Sen, Abu Abraham, and many others to the campus. I also got opportunities to travel to Finland and some European countries, South Korea, Hong Kong, etc., for study programs and to participate in conferences. These travels were golden opportunities for me to learn more about the people and the world.

My yearning for higher studies continued, though I encountered many difficulties. Meanwhile, I married Sheela from Mysore, who was working in a bank, and a baby (Anand) was born. I wanted to study further in one of the best universities in the country; but that meant a hard struggle ahead. After a difficult process, finally I got admission for MA in Sociology in the Jawaharlal Nehru University (JNU), New Delhi, with a monthly stipend of Rs.190. My wife also got a transfer to her bank branch near the JNU Old Campus. We stayed in a garage in Vasant Vihar when we came to Delhi from Bangalore in 1974. Those were trying times and since then we have stayed in 11 different places in Delhi. Our present home is the twelfth. Initially we had a Rajdoot motorcycle to move around in the city. Anyway, we were determined to face our hardships and realise our dreams.

I completed MA in Sociology in two years and our second son (Suresh) was born when we were in the married students hostel on the old campus. After my post graduate degree, it took two years for my M. Phil. and another two years for Ph. D. These six years were transformative for me. Apart from attending classes and reading in the JNU Old Campus Library till midnight, I was inspired by my meetings with rebel political leaders like George Fernandes, Chandrasekhar and Jayaprakash Narayan. Then my passion was to write articles on the contemporary social issues which got published in *Blitz* and other publications.

After I took Ph. D. from the JNU, I was invited as Visiting Fellow at the South-Asia Centre, Chicago University, USA, during 1981-82. There I could interact with intellectuals and scholars and travel to different parts of USA and Canada, which made me to think that the good and positive actions taking place in America must happen in my motherland too. The Institute of Social Sciences that I set up in Delhi is in a sense the realization of that dream that I had while I was in the USA.

While we were in Chicago, my wife worked at the Hyde Park Bank and our two kids studied in the primary school near the campus. Profs. Lloyd and Susanne Rudolph were our mentors. After we returned to Delhi, my concern was the emerging socio-political situation in the country and I became an active member of the People's Union for Civil Liberties (PUCL) which was led by many inspiring leaders like V. M. Tarkunde, Kuldip Nayar, Arun Shourie, Inder Mohan and many others. When the 1984 Sikh massacre occurred, I was one of the conveners of the People's Relief Committee, working from 7 Jantar Mantar, day and night. All this time, my thought was how to be an active player to bring about positive transformation in our society.

In the late 1970s and early 80s, the terms which widely gained currency were "activism-oriented intellectuals" and "intellectually-oriented activists." Some of us, who were products of this wave or social paradigm, were in a way impatient to translate this thinking into reality. In a sense, the Institute of Social Sciences is the result of this intellectual quest. It was a reaction to the ivory-tower academic exercises and a search for social knowledge based on hard realities of society and unity of study and action. When the Institute of Social Sciences was registered in 1985, the location was F-67 Bhagat Singh Market, New Delhi 110001, which was Inder Mohan's residential flat from where the PUCL was functioning. The 35-year period from F-67 Bhagat Singh Market to 8 Nelson Mandela Road, with several regional research centres, was a long journey of struggle and achievements.

Over the years, my conviction and principle have been that if there is a will there is a way and today I have an excellent network of friends around the world from whom I have learned immensely to pursue the kind of social and intellectual activities I could involve myself in.

Democratic decentralisation is the bedrock on which the edifice of the Institute of Social Sciences has been erected. In course of time, the ISS began expanding its scope to include more areas that tied up with serious democratic concerns. In the main, these are: grassroots democracy, women's empowerment, human rights and global issues affecting humanity. While no hard-and-fast rule excludes any worthwhile area of research, advocacy, training, monitoring and public engagement, the identity of the ISS lies basically in these four areas of involvement with Panchayati Raj as its flagship programme. National leaders of various persuasions like Ramakrishna Hegde, Abdul Nazir Sab, George Fernandes, N. T. Rama Rao, Farooq Abdullah, S. K. Dey, Nirmal Mukarji, L. C. Jain and Rajni Kothari contributed to the democratic vision of the ISS.

It is a matter of pride that the Institute could associate itself with Amartya Sen, Noam Chomsky, Mahbubul Haq, Muhammad Yunus, Asma Jehangir, Bhikhu Parekh, Albie Sachs, Romila Thapar, Manmohan Singh, K. R. Narayanan and many other eminent persons. Former President of India Dr. A. P. J. Abdul Kalam gave a mission to the Institute while delivering the eighth D. T. Lakdawala Memorial Lecture at the Mavlankar Hall, New Delhi on 18 August 2010, which was a historic moment for all associated with the Institute.

According to Dr. Abdul Kalam, The Institute of Social Sciences will provide to the nation: The best practices of Panchayats across the nation may be documented and used as training material across multiple regions and languages of the nation. Multimedia documenting the profile of the best Panchayats in the nation will act as inspiration for the local youth to take up leadership roles in the future" and The Institute should emerge as a platform for consulting individual Panchayats on how they can best achieve the goals of local-level development using the existing government and non-government schemes."

When I was growing up in Kerala, C. Kesavan was the Chief Minister of Travancore-Cochin in 1950-52. He wrote an autobiography titled '*Jeevithasamaram*' (Life is a struggle) describing the trials and tribulations he underwent as he was born in a village in a backward community (Ezhava), which was considered as untouchable. The discrimination he suffered wherever he went and the unjust behaviour of elders did not stop him from reaching the highest position in the state. Why? He took life as a struggle leading to achievement.

From my early years, when I started the thinking process, I could read C. Kesavan's *Jeevithasamaram*. I have taken my life as a struggle and my motto has been, "Never give up, and look ahead".

25
THE ART OF AGEING GRACEFULLY
GENERAL (RETD.) V. N. SHARMA

All species that are born on this earth must die. Some live many years and some die early, some are sickly and some are healthy for reasons not well known. In the life span granted to us humans by fate or destiny it is unclear whether we have any control over the way we choose to live, to act, to deal with problems and obstacles that confront us or whether we function entirely on inborn instinct like that of animals and birds. The difference between us and other species is the human mind that controls our actions in addition to natural instinct. Essential bodily functions remain automatic in all living species but the human mind is beset with thoughts and desires which affect the way we act and the way we deal with others. For a long and happy life it is necessary to learn the art of living and handling the body and mind.

The human body is the finest energy machine nature has designed. No scientist or medical doctor has yet fully understood how this energy machine works or how it is controlled and by whom it is controlled. Like any machine, this too requires adequate maintenance and correction of faults by treatment as it grows older. With prolonged use it can develop faults by injury, infection, misuse or accident. The ancient Greek physician to whom the 'Oath of Hippocrates' is attributed basically enjoined all healers to swear to benefit their patients according to the best of their ability and do them no harm or injustice. Yet today many patients have little trust in their medical doctors and run from one to another seeking a number of opinions in their desire for authentic and cheap treatment. This is because some doctors have gained a poor reputation for making money by treating patients to become more dependent on medication. Many private hospitals have gained a similar reputation of greed and financial sleight at the cost of patients. Medical authorities and doctors in many nations come under the financial control of the pharmaceutical industry which must sell its expensive drugs to make huge profits at the cost of public health. It is obvious that for human beings prevention of disease is better than dependence on medical cure. Hospitals must only be visited if there is a health emergency and no other alternative.

To look after this body of ours over all the years of life that are given to us, it is necessary to keep it healthy, physically fit and mentally calm, to prevent disease and develop good immunity to disease. Many do not realize that the main control of this energy machine is by the human mind. The mind is not an organ of the body but is an ephemeral spiritual control under the supervision of the intellect. The body and mind are closely connected to mental thought processes and physical activity. If the senses feel danger the body is immediately prepared for 'fight or flight' by adrenaline and other hormones being instantly injected into the bloodstream to activate the brain, muscles and vital organs, the heartbeat is rapidly increased and lungs forced to breathe much faster. This causes damage to bodily systems if intense physical activity does not ensue. Further, the brain and mind cannot think clearly under such a physical or mental danger, anger, or fear syndrome as action is instinctive and not carefully thought out. These are natural instinctive reactions for preservation of life. But such reactions can result in serious personal harm to body structures under normal circumstances of daily human contact where foul or impolite language or aggression causes uncontrollable temper and threat of physical violence. A calm and controlled mind can help to avoid physical or mental damage.

The main need for physical and mental health is, therefore, control over the mind. This control must ensure a cool, collected and calm mind at all times. Mental thoughts display continuous pictures in the 'mind's eye'; these must be controlled to see nothing, to only see a blank. Many sayings indicate this in all religions. To keep the mind in a calm state and to prevent angry or emotional feelings, the mind must be kept involved in a semi-spiritual state by prolonged religious mental chanting, by repeated mantras, or constant 'watching the breath'. The breath is a vital life source, it must be regular and deep i. E. each breath must be drawn deep into the broad lower lungs, bearing on the diaphragm and thus expanding the stomach cavity. In the Sermon on the Mount, the Lord Jesus advised "Turn ye the other cheek" when asked how one should act when he is slapped by someone. This advice was not to meekly accept undeserved punishment but to calm the mind; then only would it be possible for the victim to clearly decide on what concerted action to take. In the Buddhist tradition the guidance is to be calm and develop love for all beings. All Hindu deities have one hand raised with the palm facing the seeker, not only to give blessings but to encourage calmness and to 'cool it'. Islam gives the example of Hazrat Ali, the son-in-law of the Holy Prophet, who was a great warrior. On the field of battle when in single combat with a selected strong enemy warrior, to decide which side was victorious between the two opposing armies, Hazrat Ali was able to throw his opponent to the ground and had his sword at the enemy's throat to win the day for his side but his opponent spat in Ali's face. Hazrat Ali wiped his face, got his opponent to stand up, retrieve his sword and give battle again. A few hours later he was able to kill the enemy and returned victor to his side. His commander threatened severe punishment and demanded an explanation for Ali's dangerous behaviour which may have caused ignominy and defeat of his army if the enemy had won the contest. Ali stated he was a soldier and not a murderer; he was remorseless in killing the enemies of his kingdom because that was his duty, though he had no hate nor had any anger for the enemy since they too did their duty to their own king; but when his opponent spat in his face Ali felt violent anger and hurt ego since he had overcome the enemy and was obviously the superior fighter. He immediately wanted to thrust his sword into the hated enemy's neck and kill; but he controlled himself with the thought that if he did this, he would be a cold-blooded murderer as he would be killing for his own hate and revenge, not for his king and country. Having cooled his mind and controlled his anger, he got his opponent to fight again and then killed for his duty to king and country. This was a fine example of non-violence, a cool collected mind in full control of the body and doing duty as desired of a soldier. The mind can be promptly calmed by watching the breath and controlling the flow to take deep breaths; this restores the mind to cool calculated thought to guide the body to correct and effective action.

Once the mind is trained to be calm with controlled emotion and steady deep thought, it achieves total fearlessness and can carry out effective guidance of the body's actions no matter what the situation. As said in the Bhagavad Geeta the human is then capable of maximum efficiency in the true direction without any concern for the results of such action as results are not under control of the individual. The immune system remains highly effective and disease is blocked. Such an individual develops an attractive aura which tends to cause others to respect and assist such a soul's journey through life and keeps the body young and supple over the years.

The human energy machine certainly requires daily maintenance and repair. This is best done by daily hard exercise consistent with mind control and high value nutrition. Good nutrition is fundamental to healthy life. We are exposed to a polluted environment and polluted food due to the financial greed of individuals who produce food and run factories as they prefer to make a 'quick buck' rather than bother about the health of others. It is necessary for us to try and keep our environment clean, breathe clean air and eat a pure simple nutritious diet. We should try and avoid becoming slaves to our taste and always eat a little less than what we desire, to prevent over-eating. The body is designed for action. Avoidance of daily, hard physical activity causes serious deterioration of health. As one gets older the need is for more attention to daily workouts, games and sports, brisk walking and jogging, in a happy environment rather than acting like a debilitated old person with bent back and balancing with the help of a stick. The spine must always be kept straight by standing and sitting 'tall' no matter what your age. The best and most scientific system of exercise is undoubtedly yoga, with special attention to pranayama, since breath is life. Yoga exercises must be initially learned from a good teacher who can correct faulty damaging techniques and is not greedy for money but charges reasonable fees; we are lucky in India to be able to access free yoga training on the television by evolved teachers like Guru Ramdev. The main stress of exercise in old age is to build steady balance of the body, carry out various stretches for flexibility of spine and do strengthening exercises against the weight of the body, such as squats and push-ups. Balancing on one leg for at least a half minute daily is essential as one gets older. When one walks or runs, only one leg is on the ground at a time, while the other is in the air while stepping forward. Most old people tend to trip and fall which may cause serious injury such as a broken hip or leg bone. This could be a death sentence since losing one's use of legs prevents normal movement and exercise besides reducing mobility and the pleasure of life in his beautiful world. There is the need for special attention to leg exercises, good balance and flexible joints. One must also learn and perfect the art of falling backwards, forwards or sideways to prevent serious injury to the lower limbs. Basically the art comprises the instinctive slapping of the ground hard with the hands to break the fall, also to tuck in the head to the chest for a backward fall to prevent a broken neck. One can learn from observing how parachutists perform a roll if they have an awkward descent on earth.

The mind must be trained to enjoy life. Enjoy the beauties of nature and the love and affection of relatives and friends. The need is to look at others, even if they are strangers, with respect and a feeling of joy, to smile rather than scowl, to feel good about yourself and to feel good about all others too. This is known as the "I am OK, you are OK" syndrome. It leads to good health and long life, to a life of grace and style. The Indian concept of "Vasudhaiva Kutumbakam" or 'the world is one family' says it all. Your attitude to all the vicissitudes of life is vital. All humans face problems and obstacles as they proceed in the journey of life, these are building blocks of high character and good conduct if overcome in the correct spirit, an attitude of 'will do' and 'can do'. A positive and confident attitude with a happy and trusting heart leads to success in your undertakings and also to easy forbearance of failure. Failure itself is always temporary and a part of the journey which, if taken 'in your stride' leads to better experience and success. Daily exercise and yoga allows complete physical control over the body, the limbs, joints, muscles and sinews. This lends grace and charm to all bodily movements, the way one walks, runs or sits. Mind control gives you the art of attractive and modulated respectful speech. Such training increases the aura of your presence, improves your vibes and enhances the chances of a long peaceful, happy life. You should examine carefully each day all the incorrect actions and transgressions made by your behaviour and resolve to correct such poor conduct and apologise or make amends to those adversely affected by your behaviour.

As stated earlier, death is axiomatic to all living species. Why then should there be a fear or horror of death? Most families never mention the word in case it brings morbid thoughts and bad luck. Such fears perhaps shorten your life, since all fear reduces immunity. Fear is a nasty and depressive thought and has its ill effect on health. You must get rid of all fear; the Afghan Pathan's greeting contains the saying "Fikkar Nishta", meaning 'get rid of fear' these being violent tribes which face injury or death daily. Our soldiers are trained to accept the possibility of death so they can carry out their duties fearlessly. The warrior's code claims direct access to Valhalla (the Old Norse warrior heaven) in case of death. To live a carefree long life with grace and health it is necessary to fearlessly face the probability of death. Our Shastras claim the soul is everlasting and never dies. This thought gives confidence to human beings to have no worries but be full of anticipation of the adventures and new experiences that await the conscience once life passes, giving one a better perspective of the mysteries of the universe and perhaps bringing one closer to God. Such thoughts alone give us humans the calm self confidence to face all future incidents, even death.

The training of the mind has a spiritual content. Watching and counting the breath, with simultaneous chanting, occupy the mind and create calm. This is meditation. All humans are beset with a big noise and myriad thoughts in the head because of the busy mind which is constantly active like a super computer always 'on the go'. It is a lifetime effort to control and reduce this noise and success is possible by constant deliberate effort. Swami Yogananda (*Autobiography of a Yogi*) stated that the mind sees a false world like an interesting film on a screen; where the actors play their part causing the audience to participate in the actor's tribulations, joys and sorrows; but it is all unreal once the film ends and a blank screen is left. The great Indian saint Ramana Maharishi of Thiruvannamalai in Tamil Nadu had said that "the real is ever present like the screen on which cinematographic pictures move, while the picture appears on it the screen remains invisible. Stop the picture and the screen will become clear. All thoughts and events are pictures moving on the screen of pure consciousness, which alone is real". Similarly the Lord Jesus instructed, "The Kingdom of Heaven lies within, seek and ye shall find it. Knock and the door shall be opened unto you". The greatest advantage of growing old gracefully is that the individual has time to learn the lessons of life, to accept with fortitude the weakening of the body and the destruction of ego when others must help to carry out even the most intimate tasks of daily routine; and above all, to improve the quality of the soul and thoughts to go to a superior existence of consciousness.

26
OLD IS GOLD
ZARINA BHATTY

Old age is often referred to as the 'the golden age' of one's life. 'Old is Gold' is also an oft-repeated phrase. But in reality, 'old' is a negative term in all languages and cultures. It refers to things that have outgrown their usefulness and are to be replaced. Human beings, like all living creatures, also grow old after going through the natural stages of childhood, youth, and finally old age – an inevitable stage of life, unless of course, one dies young.

There are two sides to the coin called old age. On one hand, it can be a pain, physically, mentally and emotionally; various disabilities creep in as one starts ageing. Fortunately, nature is kind and the disabilities do not overtake all of a sudden, but gradually and slowly, both body and mind losing their agility inch by inch. The other side of the coin depends on your attitude. One must try to accept disabilities with a sense of humour, taking them as a natural process. Alongside, if one is surrounded by empathetic near and dear ones who do the same, old age can be a joy.

Sometimes, age-related afflictions can lead to funny situations. Hearing loss is most common in old age and can lead to situational humour. For example, a while back, my granddaughter called my husband who had become hard of hearing. "*Nana, kya wahan baarish ho rahi hai?*" she asked him. ("Is it raining there?"). He replied, "*Main maalish kab karaata hoon?*" ("When do I ever get a massage?"). My granddaughter started giggling, leaving my husband most puzzled. Apparently, one can also have what is medically termed as 'discriminatory' hearing loss whereby one can hear some people fully but not others. I suffer from this kind of hearing problem. When I am watching television or am in a group, I miss out on a particular speaker's conversation and keep nudging the person next to me to repeat what was said. It leads to a lot of irritation in the others. "Oh Mummy/ Nannu/ Auntie, why don't you get hearing aids?". I have been resisting them for some years as most of my friends who are using them are not quite happy. It was only recently that I finally decided to appease the young ones and get a pair.

On enquiry, I found that prices ranged between INR 50000 to several lakhs, depending not only on their efficacy but also on how successfully they could be hidden. The salesman gleefully spread out a number of hearing aids for me to choose from. "Here madam, you take this one, it will fit into your ears so well that no one will be able to guess your age", he said. To his annoyance, I asked, "Would it also hide my greying hair and wrinkles?"). But madam, I think you should dye your hair, then with this device tucked in your ears you will look ten years younger," he replied, displaying a typically insensitive attitude that people have when it comes to older women. "Madam, it will only cost you one lakh, it has a tiny loop which goes round the ears and I shall try to make it as invisible as possible", he continued, still insisting that I should hide my age, this to my utmost annoyance. Eventually, I settled on a pair costing a handsome amount of one lakh rupees and had it fitted into my eighty-seven years old fragile ears. It is another story that I dropped one of them only a few days later and there went my hard-earned fifty thousand rupees.

When faced with such a situation, one will certainly blurt out "Old age is a pain". But as I have earlier pointed out, one can also look back on the positive aspects of old age, such as the huge stock of learning and experiences gathered over the years - good, bad, happy, and sad. The carefree days of childhood, the innocent friendships made; the physical agility and of course good hearing too, the large number of people one had met and interacted with, from various regions, religions and cultures, black, yellow and white people, infant, young and old; the travels within one's own country and even across national borders, the variety of languages, music and dances one has heard, seen and enjoyed and above all the variety of cuisines one has tasted (I am a foodie). After all, what is life if not a huge bundle of experiences? So old age is not just a pain, it is also to be cherished because the longer one lives, the wider the range of experiences becomes.

When I look back and remember the exuberance of my youth, the joys of learning, professional achievements, the priceless feeling of holding my first college degree and my first pay packet in my hands, the sense of economic independence, the excitement of my first embrace with my lover, the sweetness of our first kiss, and the unadulterated joy of my first born and other children, of so many more moments of happiness and of sadness too, like losing my parents and the persisting grief of having lost my husband. The age-related aches and pains melt away when one starts counting the numerous blessings that Nature and God have bestowed upon my family over the years. As the poet says, "*Ginwaun toh ginwa na sakun*" (So many that they are impossible to count, even if I try).

As mentioned earlier, in almost all languages and cultures, the word 'old' refers to things that have become redundant. However, I must point out the slight difference in attitude when it comes to Asian societies, India particularly. Here, economic realities dictate that nothing is discarded, rather, most things are recycled. The modern concept of recycling, which is talked about a great deal nowadays, was always there in our culture. I remember how my mother used to make colourful 'razais' (comforters} with old sarees and 'ghararas' (flared skirts).

In the same way old persons were revered, not sneered at or considered useless. They were respected and made to feel useful. For instance, chewing 'paan' (Betel leaves stuffed with finely cracked betel nuts) was a habit of both the old and the young in Uttar Pradesh. Old ladies, who were not very mobile, had the task of cracking betel nuts, and making 'gilori' covers out of used paper. 'Gilori' is the word used for the conical, ready-to-eat 'paan'. Betel leaf presented to visitors in hand-made 'gilori' covers. I remember my grandmother feeling gainfully engaged and important as she went about this task. Similarly, the cook would be instructed to give her peas for shelling. Her advice was sought on menus, recipes and on the correct methods of cooking family dishes. Educated older people would be requisitioned to help with the grandchildren's homework, thus helping young parents. Thus the experiences and wisdom of old persons was utilised and appreciated, and they were well looked after within the structure of the joint family, which was the norm, rather than the exception. Come to think of it, old age continues to be revered in India, although economic changes and the advent of technology are posing practical difficulties in caring for elderly persons.

Fact is, ageing is an indelible fact of life. I find solace in my past, when I was in full control of my mind and body. Now as an octogenarian, I am losing control (gradually, thank God) over my movements. I have difficulty in walking, bathing, in keeping my body balanced when I stand up and even in changing clothes. Time and again, I end up putting my foot into the wrong side of the 'salwar' (pyjamas) in spite of checking several times before wearing it.

I also wear my shirts back to front. I did none of this before but then I have never been eighty-seven before. Interestingly, I checked with my friend next door who is my age and he confessed that he too had to wear and remove his shirt several times before he could get it right. Another embarrassing problem is that I drop food on my clothes while eating. My daughter says, "All mummy's shirts and sarees have her stamp - i.e., food droppings". She remarked that her mother-in-law's sarees have similar stamps. I think our necks shrink as we age and with the decreased distance, we end up dropping bits of food. I am glad my children take this affliction with a pinch of humour. In a film I saw, an old man would drop things on the floor including cups and plates, till the daughter-in-law got tired of losing her crockery and got paper plates for him. The five-year-old grandson found it fascinating that the grandfather was using different plates every mealtime. He gleefully tells his father that he would get similar plates for him when he grew old. The son and daughter-in-law realised that they did not have to be intolerant of age-related infirmities; it was only a matter of time when they would be old too. This story reminds me of a simple but very apt verse. "*Jo jaake naa aye who jawani dekhi, aur jo aa ke naa jaye who budhapa dekha*". ("I have experienced youth, which will never return, and old age which will never go away".)

Another very common affliction of elderly persons lies in the change of signature. My husband would practice his signature assiduously before signing a cheque and it would still not match the original. This is happening to me too. I cannot do mental calculations any more, although I used to be very good in Mathematics. I had a distinction in High School and was teased by my classmates for being the teacher's pet.

Loss of memory is another gift of old age, particularly when it comes to numbers and names. Sometime ago I met a friend after many years, in Connaught Place, New Delhi. She hugged me and whispered in my ears, 'I am Safia, in case you have forgotten my name". It was so thoughtful of her because I had actually forgotten her name. These days I keep myself amused by discovering my newest age-related affliction every morning. One can play a guessing game with fellow octogenarians by sharing each other's age-related experiences. For example, the other day I asked my neighbour what he was reading. He could not remember the title of the book but he said he was enjoying it. I fully empathised with him. I too like reading and often forget the title or the name of the author, but I do not fret about it. After all, as the saying goes, "What's in a name?". My days are full of surprises these days. This morning I discovered, or rather was made to realise by my domestic help that I was losing connection between thinking, planning and execution.

"Memsahib, I had asked you to put onions also on the shopping list but you forgot", she said. "Of course I did, in fact I remember writing two kilos, so that they last longer", I replied. But when I checked the list, onions were not on it. The mismatch between thought and action is happening more and more frequently as I am collecting years, and is becoming a cause of irritation for those around me. I give credit to my maid for dealing with me with patience. But such qualities are becoming rare these days and there are good reasons for that. Life is so fast-paced, no one has the time to be patient.

Human longevity has increased. Those of us in our seventies or eighties today are the first generation of elderly persons to live so long. This has created new issues both in families and societies. I have no doubt that the majority of young persons would like to take care of their parents, but they face many practical problems. Science and technology have brought about tremendous changes not only in their aspirations but as a consequence, in their lifestyles and even in their thought processes. There are so many more avenues of work and ways of earning money. Alongside, the desire for affluence and the drive to live more comfortable lives has become paramount. Exposure to advanced societies, new means of entertainment, possibilities of national and international travel, etc., are creating new aspirations. Cinema, television and the Internet have created new needs. Facebook, Twitter, etc., keep youngsters busier than ever. To meet the demands of modern living, husband and wife both need to work. This may entail long hours of commuting, late working hours, tackling competition, factors that in turn cause stress and frustration. Two salaries are becoming essential. There is a huge cost of living, with maids and tutors, exorbitant school fees and skyrocketing rents, especially in urban areas. Those with moderate incomes are forced to live in smaller dwellings, where privacy is compromised, leading to anger. When I was growing up, a separate room for each child was not considered necessary. Older persons did not mind sharing a room with grandchildren.

I decided to do an informal survey and talked to a number of friends, relatives, neighbours and former colleagues in their seventies and eighties. I found many common problems, specially related to physical decline, like loss of memory, hearing impairment, difficulty in walking, progressively losing teeth, dementia and even Alzheimer's and Parkinson's disease. Medical science has found treatments for many of these illnesses, but these are partial, and their efficacy varies a great deal from individual to individual. Besides, most of these medical solutions, such as organ replacement, hearing aids, dentures, teeth transplants, etc., are very expensive and beyond the reach of even lower middle-class persons, leave alone the poor. Although health insurance is available, it is very inadequate. Government services are scarce and do not cover expensive medicines and procedures. Private health facilities are so costly that they are limited to the rich. Although non-governmental organisations (NGOs) like Guild of Service are doing remarkable work, they cannot cover the entire country. Having weighed all the pros and cons, here is what I would like to say in conclusion.

The evening of life also has its advantages. Firstly, elderly persons have all the time at their disposal, to use it as they please. No sleepless nights, changing nappies and feeding babies; no waking up in the wee hours to send children to school; no seeing to children's homework; no taking care of old parents or in- laws, no organising their meals or giving them medicines on time, etc., For working women, in addition to domestic responsibilities, there is the stress of reaching office on time, meeting professional targets, fighting for promotions, etc. In old age these responsibilities have been fulfilled, the children have grown. So one can sleep as late as one desires, read the books one didn't ever have time for and maybe even learn something new, like playing an instrument. There are many additional joys, like grandchildren to play with, time to read each and every section of the newspaper and generally to do as one pleases. When I was young, I had so many responsibilities – as a mother, as a daughter-in-law and as a teacher. There was never any time to indulge in fiction and my reading was strictly work-related. Now I can read fiction to my heart's delight. I can also watch all the television programs I wish to, especially live tennis matches.

I have even dared to write a book at the age of eighty and am planning another one too. It is a competition now between my planned book and myself. Will I complete the book first or complete my life term first? Let's see. Frankly, it does not matter either way. I have won most competitions in life and am quite content to lose now.

27
YOUNG FOREVER
ARUNA VASUDEV

Ageing gracefully is not by any means an easy process. You don't realise you don't have the physical energy and even the mental energy required for doing all that you have done easily through your life. And suddenly that becomes a nuisance as many thoughts cross your mind about all that you wish to carry on doing and don't have the strength to continue doing any longer. Principally it is the physical energy that has diminished, not the mental!

You think you can carry on writing, working, going here and there to listen to music, watch a dance performance or a play, go and see the new film or an art exhibition you wish to see, friends you want to meet, talks you want to listen to - or participate in – write articles or work on a book.... As you set out to do any of these things, you suddenly stop and think – No, I'll go and meet this friend, have a coffee or a drink, and just relax.

It doesn't always work! You force yourself to get back to work, to go to the film or any of the above performances you need to see that you have to write about, or participate in a discussion where you have to speak, or – so many activities you have been engaged in throughout your life which have given you so much satisfaction but suddenly the energy to participate in them seems to have vanished.

That is very troubling and requires will and determination to slow down and take it easy! But, do not give up. To do all that gave you so much energy, excitement – and inspiration to live a magically full and exciting life: why should you give it up? No, as long as you are up and about and using your mind, you can carry on as before without any hindrances. The physical and mental energy does not disappear as long as you yourself don't give up.

The only thing I have given up is travelling alone. That does bother me and I will only travel if I have a companion. At the end of 2019, I was invited to the jury of a film festival in China – a beautiful island, and I loved the idea of going but I told them, "No. Very sorry but I cannot travel alone." As this was on an island off the coast of China, to get there you had to fly to Beijing, and change planes. Having done that and more for so, so many years of my life I even asked my self, "What is the matter? Why can't you do that?" But my mind said, "NO". Then a young filmmaker friend of mine said she would come, pay her own fare, if she could share a room with me. I was delighted; the Festival agreed immediately and we went to this beautiful island where I had one of the most enjoyable experiences of my life.

That was just under a year ago. Other possibilities also came up but then the lockdown due to the Covid 19 pandemic started and that was the end of travel, and even of any work that involved moving outside your home. Life changed radically. I went back to painting and carried on with it daily for a few months when all of a sudden it hit me that the life I had lived from the start, had come to an end. So you go through a period of depression, telling yourself that you have to accept your age, that you no longer have the strength, the energy, the will power to carry on as you did for decades. But in fact, that is not the case. So many people across the world have carried on spectacularly, with their work, their interest in life, their will to continue doing all that they want to. It is quite inspiring to learn about that.

But one has to accept the fact that physically there is a lowering of energy; but as long as the mind is clear, one can carry on and on! Not engaged in too many physical activities but certainly activities of the mind. Although I have a friend who, over the age of 80, is still playing tennis! That, of course, is exceptional but the mind does not age. It may slow down a bit but as long as the will and the desire to continue, is there, one can carry on.

Physical energy is not required to continue writing, teaching, learning, reading, discussing ideas, coming up with new ideas for what can be done. So much of one's being depends on the mind, and the mind does not necessarily age as the body does. Ideas keep coming to your head as one keeps on reading, dreaming, following up on things that have interested you in your life.

There is a time when one feels "enough". You want to stop thinking, doing, running around – just give up and sit at home with the young ones in the family, playing with them, occasionally meeting up with friends, and doing nothing. But when you have been active your whole life, that doesn't work. Of course, one wants time to spend with family and the few friends still around, but this can lead to a very low state of mind. So to get back to being as active as one has been all one's life, leads to a new energy and that is very very important.

All my life I have worked. I made a decision when I was in my last year of school – and that was a long, long time ago, in 1952 – that I would definitely work. While in college, in Delhi, I started doing small, odd jobs with radio and television, went with the generosity of my supportive parents to Europe to study French and German – two languages I really wanted to learn – then came back to Delhi and discovered television. I became fascinated by television and managed to find small jobs with TV – which was then just a couple of hours twice a week from Delhi – and then life opened up for me. I went with my parents to New York where my father was posted, took a short but intensive course in film and television and then my life began. I didn't like New York, surprisingly enough. I went to the great Film School in Paris and then it is a long story.

But a very extraordinary and exciting and fulfilling story. Years of learning, working, travelling and then - No more Paris

– or Europe – but back in India where I wanted to be. Then first making documentary films, then writing, then starting an international quarterly on Asian cinema – *Cinemaya* – which ran for 25 or so years, then an Asian Film Festival in Delhi – Cinefan in 1999 – which immediately became such a major event that I ended up handing it to Neville Tuli and Osians about five years later because to collect so much financial support was impossible! Along the way, in 1991, we had created NETPAC – Network for the Promotion of Asian Cinema – which is now an established international institution.

It is a long story! When I decided I did not really wish to continue with such intense but hugely satisfying work, I decided to stay home and started an annual Festival of Buddhist Film, Art and Philosophy which is still continuing off and on. The last edition was last year but this year, like so much else, it was impossible. One can only wait and see what the future will bring.

What will it bring? Does anyone know?

That is life, and that is the way we have to carry on to an unknown future. That is what one has to live with, and the philosophy of Buddhism helps enormously in coping with such a confusion-riddled world.

28

Growing Old So That the Best Is Yet to Be

Pascal Alan Nazareth

In my long life, 35 years of which I have spent abroad in diverse countries while in the Indian Foreign Service, I have seen many tumultuous events, both tragic and brutal as also inspiring and mysterious. In the 25 years of retirement thereafter, I have suffered two personal tragedies and been deeply affected by both of them. All these experiences, as also the valuable maxims I learnt since my youth, have contributed to my slow but steady evolution from youthful exuberance and the urge for immediate action and results to a more measured pace of life and thoughtful, well-considered action.

During the eleven years I spent in my grandparents' home in Mangalore when I studied at St. Aloysius College Mangalore, Aunt Brice, was my loving, caring and constant guide. She taught me to be respectful to elders and unselfish in my ways. One evening when I joyfully recounted a prank my classmates and I had played on our Hindi teacher she gently reminded me that some years earlier my father had taught in the same school and asked, "Would you have rejoiced over a similar prank on him by his students?". This impacted on me so deeply that thereafter I never took part in such pranks. For Christmas 1946, my parents had gifted me a new silk shirt. My cousin Joe Mathias was not as fortunate. Coffee prices were very low that year and his coffee planter father could not afford to give Christmas gifts to his seven children. So Aunt Brice suggested that I lend Joe my linen bush shirt for attending Christmas Mass. As I was very fond and proud of it, I refused to do so. She then gently pointed out that Christmas was not about new clothes and gifts but emulating the Infant Jesus, who chose to be born in a cow shed rather than a palace and by doing so taught us to be humble and unselfish. So I reluctantly complied with her request. Joe's great joy over this unexpected kindness clearly proved the great worth of her advice. Some weeks later, when there was much commotion over an alleged theft of her mother's gold bangles, she intervened stating, "It is always better to light a candle than curse the darkness", calmly enquired who had last handled these bangles and within the next hour was able to locate them. I have always remembered and practiced these maxims of Aunt Brice.

Fr. Stanley Coelho, Asst. Headmaster of St. Aloysius College moulded my youthful views on studies, student hobbies, religion, and spirituality. He urged me to read as much as possible particularly literary classics, poetry compilations and biographies of great leaders, to participate in sports and strive to excel in one of them and spend weekends in gardening or hiking so as to discover "the wonder and beauty of nature". He clarified the difference between religion and spirituality, that the latter was the nourishing of one's soul and ensuring its growth, and therefore was more important than the former. He also stressed the need to be loyal and proud of India as it was our mother land, a prime "Mother Civilization" of the world.

For Christmas 1949 he presented me with a bookmark with 'A Boy's Prayer'. It read as under:

I pray whatever wrong I do,
I will never say what is not true;
Be willing at my task each day,
And always honest in my play.

Make me unselfish with my joys,
And generous to the other boys;
And kind and helpful to the old,
And prompt to do what I am told.

Bless every one I love, and teach
Me how to help and comfort each;
Give me the strength right living brings,
And make me good in little things"

I made this prayer my "Mission Statement" from the day I received it. I still have this bookmark with me.

When my grandfather Pascal D'Souza's life was ebbing away on June 23, 1951, my grandmother, other members of the family and I were gathered around his bed praying for him when his breathing finally stopped. This was the first time I witnessed death at the very moment it happened. A remarkable phenomenon occurred at that moment. All the poultry which my grandfather had lovingly fed every day when in good health, cackled loudly as if they were seeing his soul depart and were mourning his departure. From that day I have been convinced there is a close but invisible connection between the physical and spiritual worlds.

In December 1952, while doing my two-year Pre-University course at Government Arts College in Cuddapah where my father was the District Judge, I witnessed the mass upsurge of grief and anger when news was received of Sri Potti Sriramulu's death following his long fast for the creation of Andhra Pradesh. As this new state came into being on October 1, 1953, I realized for the first time the potency of non-violent struggle and its self-suffering component, which Gandhi had advocated and practiced.

After completing my three-year Economics (Honours) course at Loyola College, Madras, I appeared for the Indian Administrative Sevice /Indian Foreign Service examinations in September 1957. I was called for the 'Personality Test' in February 1958, and was fairly confident of being selected - but was not. Deeply dejected, I decided not to appear for this examination again, but my deeply religious father urged me to do so and said, "Alan, we can see only up to the horizon. God sees beyond. He undoubtedly has something better in store for you next year". So I reluctantly appeared for this examination again. My father's prophetic words came true as I was selected for the Indian Foreign Service! I have therefore always remembered my father's words and often drawn inspiration and solace from them.

At my first post in the Embassy of India at Tokyo, I witnessed the distinguished Air Chief Marshal Subroto Mukherjee arrive in Tokyo as Chief Guest on Air India's inaugural Jet flight on November 8, 1960, and receive an impressive ceremonial welcome, but die the same night because Japanese *sashimi* stuck in his throat, and make a solemn return to India in a coffin! This was a stark reminder of Thomas Gray's 'Elegy in a Country Graveyard'

The boast of Heraldry, the pomp of power,
and all that beauty, all that wealth ever gave,
Await alike the inevitable hour.
The paths of glory lead but to the grave.

It was also at the Embassy of India in Tokyo that I first met the shipping magnate Jayanti Dharma Teja at the height of his wealth and power, and just five years later dealt with him as a fraudster and fugitive from justice in the US, Costa Rica, and the UK from where he was extradited to India. This was stark vindication that "Honesty is the best Policy".

At the Embassy of India in Rangoon, my residence was spacious and well furnished but dark and gloomy inside because of many leafy trees close to it. So, I had their branches trimmed. Soon thereafter my wife, who was expecting our first child became seriously sick and in the next four weeks she and the baby almost died. Amazingly all their ailments ceased when, as advised by a Burmese neighbour, I made an offering of three bottles of gin and six cakes to the Tree Spirits' whom I had angered by trimming the branches of the trees in which they lived. This has strengthened my belief that we humans live in a world inhabited by spirits which can harm us if their abodes are intruded upon.

During the three years I spent in West Africa, I witnessed or learnt at first hand of incredible brutalities in Ghana and Liberia.

These revealed the nadir to which hate filled humans can sink. But in the 8 years I spent thereafter in Latin America, the US & Britain I have seen deeply moving works of love and humanitarian and spiritual service by Mother Theresa's Missionaries of Charity, Corporate Angels, Red Cross and Hindu, Buddhist, Christian and Jewish meditation centres. All these have left deep negative and positive impressions on me.

However what has impacted me most deeply are the two personal tragedies I have experienced: the loss of my younger daughter Seema in 1999, and my younger brother John in 2014. Both were deeply painful and shattering in their effect and took me many months to recover from. The silver linings to these tragedies were that the former taught me that deep sorrow could be eased by sublimating it into humanitarian service and spiritual self-transformation. I did the former after the loss of my daughter and the latter after the loss of my brother.

A year after my daughter passed away, I set up an endowment in her name in which I invested what was her share in my estate. This endowment annually provides scholarships to bright and poor girl students and financial assistance to institutions in various parts of India providing shelter, education and vocational training to them. Among these is Guild of Service's Rahat Ghar in Kashmir.

In the months after my brother passed away, I read many books on Advaita and modern scientific research in brain science, DNA and mysticism fields such as Michael Talbot's *Mysticism and the New Physics*, Paul Davies' *The Cosmic Blue Print*' and Francis Collins' *Language of God*.

These have convinced me that all of creation, whether animate or inanimate are manifestations of the Creator, of his infinite intelligence and energy, his supreme all-pervading consciousness and cosmic master plan. God is not the many images that are made of Him/ Her and worshipped but the eternal, supremely intelligent and powerful Cosmic Energy ("Maha Shakti") which pervades and sustains the entire universe, in which every object, movement and activity, whether it is the sun that shines, the bird that sings, the flower that blooms or the child that is conceived is a manifestation of this Energy. Based on these thoughts and beliefs I composed a "Prayer to the Divine Spirit" in early 2016. It has been my daily prayer ever since:

Eternal and Almighty Divine Spirit,
I firmly believe that thou, the Creator of the whole Universe,
With its millions of stars and hundreds of galaxies,
And the exact laws and balance of forces
That keep them all in their proper orbits,
Are here within me, as the Divine Spark of Life and Energy.
That it is Thou who makes my heart to beat,
My lungs to breathe and the blood to flow,
Through every part of me, every moment of the day.
I beseech thee to fill my soul, my mind and my heart,
With thy Divine Presence,
To cleanse them of all impurity, hatred, fears and resentments
To enlighten my mind,
strengthen my will and self confidence
And assist me in resisting all temptations,
So that I will always be a good reflection of
Your Divine Presence within me.
Bless me and protect me Eternal and Almighty Divine Spirit.

This prayer gives me much spiritual comfort and mental composure at age 84 as I await the Divine summons and prepare myself for "the Best that is yet to be". Meanwhile I spend much time reading, listening to music and in gardening where I focus on tending my orchid collection.

29
AGEING GRACEFULLY
DR. SAROJA VAIDYANATHAN

Ageing is inevitable. That is the law of nature and change is the only permanent thing in this world. I have played many roles in my personal life daughter, sister wife, daughter in law, mother, mother-in-law, grandmother and great-grandmother. In my professional life, I have been and still am a Bharatanatyam exponent, a teacher, a choreographer, an author an institutional builder and administrator.

Life has been like a kaleidoscope and with each role a myriad of experiences have coloured my life and left lasting impressions on me. But I would definitely like to dwell on my interaction with the young which has rejuvenated me so much that I wear my 80 + years lightly. As one grows older, finding new companions becomes difficult because those of one's own age are beset with health problems, or have passed on.

I found whole new friends among the young who come to learn the art from me. We of course like children because they are innocent, truthful, and cute. But I find that my batteries are recharged when I am with young people like my students, my granddaughters, my young admirers. There could be many reasons for my affinity with the young. One major factor is that the younger generation is far more accommodating and they try hard not to be judgemental with respect to physical appearance. They accept you the way you are…walking slowly with a bent back, supported by a stick, slightly blind with cataract etc. And this is reflected in the ways that differently-abled sections of society today are being given opportunities to develop. This attribute helps unite minds as we go beyond physicalities. And if we are able to extend that to thought processes, we become very accommodating ready to mingle anywhere and everywhere!

The young are ever ready to laugh at you and at themselves like "*Oh … You don't know even these*" or "*How stupid of me*". Aren't these good reminders for us to shed our ego, about our image of ourselves when we were young. A good reality check for us which can help us loosen up and develop.

Many things are changing fast, and we need to quickly unlearn what we knew earlier. These young outside-the-classroom teachers impart relevant information on modern habits, language and technology to name a few, which keeps us in pace with the times. It is a constant reminder that we need to reinvent ourselves if we are to be relevant. As I said change is the only permanent thing and we need to change ourselves in how we think, how we function. Before the Covid pandemic, I had always imparted my knowledges and skill sets of Bharatnatyam face to face with my students in the classroom. But with the need for social distancing, I learnt whole new skill sets. With the help of my granddaughters, I learnt to negotiate through webinars, and zoom calls. I learnt to structure my classes to fit into the new virtual framework.

Age takes its toll on our memory and many-a-time we forget very recent instances, repeat conversations (much to the agony of the younger lot). So playing brain games, engaging in general knowledge Q&A with them, partaking in discussions of news is a must to jog the brain besides developing a connect with the youth. And when they see you as a contemporary "young-at-heart" kind, they are willing to cross the bridge to connect with your experiences and ideas.

I like to share my knowledge with them and in-depth understanding of astrology, astronomy, scriptures, rebirth with its relevance and practicality to their lives. This often endears me to them as interaction is a two-way process.

All the above are learnings of my life as a family person who has seen, shared and experienced life right from my grandparents to my great grandchildren. Every little aspect of life is a parable with a hidden meaning that you can unravel for your own benefit. Nothing in life, I feel, happens without a purpose.

One more example of what has affected my attitude to life and ageing is plant life (including micro-agriculture) like growing small rosebushes, greeneries, fruits, and vegetables. The mind is constantly at work appreciating when it grows well and wondering what went wrong when it did not. Today I almost understand plants and even talk to them at times or even sing shlokas while tending to them which I feel subconsciously, tends to liven up the plants! I also understand the transience of life through plants. What grows and gives pleasure dies one day, but it comes back in a new avatar. How reassuring this message is.

To cut a long story short, all aspects of life, the good and the bad, help us in our attitude and rejuvenate us spiritually, so that we help each other age gracefully with a feeling of belongingness and relevance to the current world!

Ageing is inevitable, but how graceful it is, is in our hands!

30

LIFE STORY INTERTWINED WITH ART OF AGEING

DR. V. SHANTA

Six decades of life as a medical professional in a unique charitable voluntary institution has been happy, unhappy, painful, bitter, frustrating but at the same time fulfilling.

What Is Fulfilling?

Vedas speak of Sat, Chit, Anandam (Existence, Knowledge, Bliss). Fulfilment is nearly but not exactly Bliss. It can only be experienced. It cannot be described. Being a medical professional is a God-given opportunity. Medicine is inseparable from service, humanity and love. Medical College and teachers taught me basic art of medicine and to follow the basic tenets of oath of Hippocrates and service to humanity.

I constantly reminded myself of great teachers and inspirational quotes which to a great extent charted the course of my life: "Action is thy duty, fruit is not thy concern", the vital premise of the Bhagavad Geeta and the inspirational lines from the Gitanjali by Rabindranath Tagore, "Give me strength never to disown the poor, or bend your knees before insolent might".

In meeting obstacles, one needs perseverance and commitment. It is important to learn from inspirational teachings and thoughts of great people, of achievers, to learn to accept your work as prayer, to accept failure as a challenge, to perceive your workplace as a temple and try to forget and forgive. There are no greater human traits than forgiveness and tolerance.

What makes one to continue despite obstacles? This will be possible only when one feels totally integrated with one's work, it becomes part of you – the two become inseparable.

Ageing, Fear of Ageing and Mortality

Ageing and mortality are inevitable, they are realities and have to be accepted as such.

It is futile to be afraid of them.

I quote from Omar Khayyam:

The Moving Finger writes; and, having writ,
Moves on: nor all thy Piety nor Wit
Shall lure it back to cancel half a Line,
Nor all thy Tears wash out a Word of it.

For one to get rid of fear of ageing, approaching ageing and death without fear, one needs rational thinking. It depends on one's attitude to life, way of life. One should plan one's future based on circumstances and environment. Fear is not the answer. Fear and apprehension cannot be shared nor measured. They have to be faced alone. The degree of fear or apprehension depends on the cause of the fear. Fear of ageing or of mortality will depend on one's attitude to life and way of life.

Great philosophers and thinkers, spiritual leaders have spent their life time to find an answer or a solution The Pavamana mantra from the Brhadaranyaka Upanishad is very inspiring:

Lead me from Darkness to Light
From Unreal to Real
From Mortality to Immortality.

Every individual has a duty to oneself, to one's family, to the work or profession you are involved in, to the community around you. A life well-lived in harmony at home, and work place, in service to the community around you, with a feeling that you have done your best, one of content, can be helpful as one grows older.

Dr. Abdul Kalam said, "You can make your Destiny".

Think less of yourself and more of what you have done or what you can do. There is still time. Plan your future. Introspection can help you to plan your future.

31
AGE OF OPPORTUNITIES
MURLIDHAR C. BHANDARE

"We don't grow older, we grow riper," said the famous painter, Pablo Picasso. The paintings Picasso produced in his final years reflect the many styles he had embraced throughout his life. As artists gather experience, contents of their art get richer and expressions get matured.

This observation is also true of all human beings—scientists, teachers, lawyers, statesmen, even ordinary men and women. In 2019, Germany-born American scientist John B. Goodenough, 97, won the Nobel Prize in Chemistry. Justice Y. V. Chandrachud, who served as the Chief Justice of India for a record term of more than seven years, passed away at the age of 88. Justice V. M. Tarkunde, considered the 'father of the civil liberties movement', lived more than 94 years. Among lawyers, Ram Jethmalani, one of India's well-known lawyers and a former union minister, died at the age of 95. An all-time great jurist, Nani Palkhivala died at the age of 82. V. S. Achyuthanandan, former Chief Minister of Kerala, is still active in politics at the age of 96. In the field of social service, Vimla Kaul, a retired English teacher, now 83, is teaching children in the slums of Delhi.

It is true that with one's age advancing, body organs begin to degenerate and one's energy diminishes. Vision becomes less distinct; hearing gets impaired; bones lose density, teeth fall and wrinkles appear on the skin. However, one gets richer in experience and wiser in perception.

I retired from active professional life at the age of 85, after serving all three wings of democracy - judiciary, legislature and executive. I served the Judiciary as an advocate for over sixty-five years, during which twice I was elected the President of the Supreme Court Bar Association. I was a member of the Parliament (Rajya Sabha) for 14 years and the Governor of Odisha for five years and a half. I travelled to all states and union territories of India and to almost all major countries spread over all continents and represented India in different UN bodies.

As I take a trip down memory lane, my past comes alive. Watching the performances of great artistes in my childhood, accompanying my father to Gandhiji's prayer meetings at different places in Mumbai and witnessing the entry of Dalits led by Babasaheb Ambedkar to our family temple at Thakurdwarin 1936 - all these and several other experiences are indelibly etched in my memory.

Pleasant memories often rush to my mind, creating sweet sensations. I remember how Sunanda and I pined to meet each other in the early years of our love. I used to take a bus from Flora Fountain to Mahim, and Sunanda waited for me at the bus stop. We would then walk on the beach holding each other's hand. One day, we decided to take ice cream and got down at Worli where there was a factory of Kwality Ice Cream. I gave her a spoonful of ice cream from my spoon and she gave me a spoonful from hers. I had a feeling as if our two lips came together, a feeling of immense joy. I also remember meeting Sunanda at Matheran, where she had gone with her friends. As I missed the connecting toy train, I had to walk all the way up the hill, where she was waiting for me. For two days, we had all the time exclusively to ourselves. Our true love never ended. It is said that those who love deeply never grow old; they may die of old age, but they die young.

Sunanda had 5 Cs – character, calibre, compassion, courtesy, and common sense. She also combined 3 Is – independence, integrity, and industry. She had inherited 3 Ps—pleasantness, patience and politeness from her father. One of the most popular

Judges of her time, she used to take final decisions on about a dozen cases every day.

Age gives a person a sense of accomplishment and fulfilment. Organising a community camp in a fisherman's village called Usarni near Dahanu in my college days was indeed an achievement. For days, we, a group of students including girls from different colleges of Mumbai, lived in the camp and along with villagers built a road that would connect the village to the main road. On the last day, about 20 villagers, whom I had not seen before, came to take part in the road construction. When I asked them why they did not come earlier, they lowered their heads and said that they were Harijans. They could not come and work with upper caste people. Then I was shocked to find that Harijans had not been invited to the evening's farewell dinner. I left the place without eating.

In the initial days of my practice, the agitation of Marathi-speaking people for a separate state gathered momentum. On November 21, 1955, about one lakh people gathered at the Flora Fountain, to stage a protest. To disperse the crowd, the police opened fire, killing a number of people. The cause of death was to be decided by the Coroner's Court, which consisted of the Judge as well as the Jury. I appeared for three of the martyrs. The Deputy Commissioner of Police gave evidence to the effect that the police had to open fire because some protesters were pelting stones. When my turn came to cross-examine him, I asked him how many protestors were pelting stones. He said over a hundred. "Where did they get the stones in and around Flora Fountain?", I asked him. He had no answer. Flora Fountain is a main square where there was no trace of stones. I summed up before the Jury, "If you believe what the Deputy Commissioner has told you, it would not be Flora Fountain, it would be Flora Mountain." The Jury gave its verdict that the firing was illegal, excessive and indefensible. The verdict gave me immense joy.

I also derived profound joy from winning a case in favour of slum dwellers of Mumbai who were deprived of electricity as they were staying in unauthorised huts. I argued that Right to Life under Article 21 of the Constitution includes right to light, air and water. The court accepted my argument, which benefitted about 25 lakh slum dwellers.

I shall also recount an interesting election case known as Invisible Ink Case, which was discussed in almost every household in the country. In the 1971 Parliamentary elections, Balraj Madhok, the Jan Sangh candidate from South Delhi Parliamentary constituency, lost to the Congress candidate, Shashi Bhushan. Madhok alleged in his election petition that thousands of ballot papers had been chemically treated and the symbol of the Congress candidate was mechanically stamped by using an invisible ink. As a result, the mark put at the time of polling disappeared after a few days and the stamp marked on the ballot paper earlier emerged. I won the case for Shashi Bhushan first in the Delhi High Court and then in the Supreme Court. The three-Judge Bench of Justice K. S. Hegde, Justice A. N. Grover and Justice D. G. Palekar held that the allegation was absolutely without any foundation.

The greatest advantage of ageing is the joy of spending time with grandchildren. For me, children are a world of joy. My three granddaughters — Shreya, Teesta and Ananya — have filled my life with immense joy. Shreya came to limelight for espousing the citizen's right to have freedom of expression. In 2012, she filed a Public Interest Litigation in the Supreme Court challenging the validity of Section 66A of the Information Technology Act, 2000, under which people could be placed under arrest for merely commenting or even 'liking' a post on a social networking website. Her case was argued by the eminent lawyer Soli Sorabjee before a bench comprising Justice J. Chelameswar and Justice Rohinton Nariman. Shreya won the landmark case for free speech and expression.

A great honour came her way in 2015, when the Government of India declared Shreya as one of the top 100 women achievers of the country. *Forbes India*, in its issue of February 19, 2016, described her as 'Freedom's Advocate'. She figured among the "30 under 30". Shreya has become a lawyer. To my utmost satisfaction, I find that she has imbibed the spirit of her grandmother.

My second granddaughter, Teesta, has a passion for freedom and empowerment of women. She was a brilliant student and her thesis, "Someone Else's Honor: Women as Repositories of Male Honor and Their Subsequent Vulnerability to Sexual Violence in India" was adjudged the Best Thesis in Legal Studies in Scripps College, USA in 2015. After completing Law at Warwick University, she is now back in Delhi. She is going to practice Law in Delhi. She takes interest in art management and curated her first art exhibition titled 'Voices of Women' at Safdarjung Enclave, New Delhi, March 14-19, 2020. The exhibition showcased 38 art pieces of 12 contemporary women artists.

My youngest granddaughter, Ananya, has an instinct for social service. As the environmental prefect of Vasant Valley School, she and her team had conceptualized a project for building 20 toilets for children in a slum in Delhi. The team won the first prize in an all-India competition conducted by Confederation of Commerce and Industry (CII) in Mumbai. The prize money of Rs 7 lakh was utilized for the project. She was instrumental in constructing twenty toilets for slum children. I felt happy taking a walk with Ananya, visiting the toilets. She graduated from Barnard College of Columbia University, worked briefly for UN Women, and is now back in Delhi. A good photographer, Ananya is also a poet. She wrote a touching poem on the occasion of my 90th birthday.

The three of them represent a new generation of India's aspiring young women. In their eyes, I see the passion and conviction of Sunanda. Today, Sunanda is no more. However, my son Rahul, his wife Namita, my daughter Manali, and my granddaughters have achieved great success in life. They take all care to keep me healthy, happy and active.

Old age offers plenty of opportunities to start volunteering in the field of one's choice. My dear friend Dr. V. Mohini Giri is devoting herself to the task of caring for aged women through the organisation, Guild of Service, which is celebrating its golden jubilee this year. Many war widows and destitute women are offered vocational training and care at 'Ma Dham' which the Guild has set up at Vrindavan.

The Justice Sunanda Bhandare Foundation, of which I am the Managing Trustee, provides me ample opportunity to serve the disadvantaged, discriminated and deprived women. The Foundation's chief objective is to ensure gender justice in our society. Its motto is: "The freedom to choose, the right to excel." To this end, it has embarked on a number of activities which include organising workshops and seminars, legal literacy camps, awareness drives, health check-up camps and blood donation camps. Every year, the Foundation organises the Justice Sunanda Bhandare Memorial Lecture on a theme relating to empowerment of women, children and differently-abled people. It has instituted the Annual Justice Sunanda Bhandare Award to be bestowed on a woman or an organisation displaying exemplary courage and dedication to the cause of gender justice.

The Foundation has filed a Public Interest Litigation in the Supreme Court for implementation of all the provisions of the Persons with Disabilities Act, 1995. It pursued the writ petition with perseverance for 16 years and finally in 2014, the Supreme Court passed an order directing the Centre, States and Union Territories to file status report of implementation of the Act.

I vividly remember the case of Manjula Rath, a visually impaired young lady, who despite having requisite qualifications, was deprived of a Lecturer's job due to lack of her sight. I fought her case in the Supreme Court and also led a protest march to the office of the University Grants Commission, but could not convince the UGC chairperson. Ultimately, I produced before the Supreme Court a circular of the Government of India in support of our case. I was delighted when my friend, Soli Sorabjee, who as the Attorney General at the time, conceded that Manjula Rath should get an appointment as a Lecturer in a college. She has proved herself an efficient and popular Lecturer in the Daulat Ram College for Women in Delhi.

I have been working for the deprived, discarded and marginalized sections of the society. I derive satisfaction from my humble work because I have no ego, no craving, and I never run after publicity. I believe in equality and dignity of every human being, which I have followed throughout my life. To me, nobody is high, nobody low; all are equal.

Today, I may not have all the energy which I possessed in the past. However, the energy I possess today is more than average, considering my age. I take my neck, back and knee exercises every morning, all seven days a week, and take homemade food. I read newspapers, magazines and books and write articles. I still play golf, which helps me keep fit and cheerful. I remember the words of George Bernard Shaw, who once said, "We don't stop playing because we grow old, we grow old because we stop playing."

Ageing population is increasing all over the world. With greater awareness and better healthcare facilities, mankind's longevity is increasing. At the global level, life expectancy at birth has reached 72.3 years. In 2019, there were 703 million persons aged 65 years or over. This number is projected to double to 1.5 billion in 2050. Globally, the number of persons aged 80 years or older nearly tripled between 1990 and 2019, growing from 54 million to 143 million; it is projected to triple again between 2019 and 2050 to reach 426 million.

With increasing longevity, mankind's active life is getting longer. An ageing population is not considered a burden on society; rather it should be an asset. A world of opportunities awaits those seniors who can contribute to society's prosperity in a meaningful way.

32
GRACE OF AGEING
SUBHASHINI ALI

"Growing old gracefully". Writing about this, I had thought, would be simple: so many women that I knew, that I had grown up admiring, had glided into old age with dignity, grace and beauty. To write about them would be simple. Just a matter of jogging my brain and bringing out some old photographs.

I sat down to write towards the end of last month and an image far removed from all those beautiful, gracious and dignified ladies came before me with such force that everything else, all those ladies and their grace, dignity and beauty, faded.

It was the image of a grieving woman, her face wrinkled and scarred with long years of hard work and humiliation, now mirroring unbearable sorrow and torment. The image of M's mother, the image of one whose own identity has now merged with that of her beloved dead daughter, the Hathras victim.

That image that haunts me still is that of a woman who is not old. She is, perhaps, in her late fifties but the harsh realities of her life and now the unbearable blow that she has suffered has ravaged her face and bent her back significantly. The long and tortuous path to justice that awaits her will certainly add to this process. And, if at the end of it, justice continues to elude her, her family and her dead daughter, the consequences are unimaginable. Growing old with grace and dignity is denied to her by her birth, by the poverty and labour that have been her inheritance, and by the terrible blows dealt to her by the cruel circumstances of her daughter's death.

It was that image that tore apart the comfortable cocoon of my contemplation of women growing old very differently, in beauty and grace. Their images had multiplied over the years, images that had not only brought joy in their viewing and remembering but which also held out the possibility of many like them emerging - the possibility and the privilege of others becoming like them. The privilege is significant: entering old age, beautiful, gracious and dignified, but it is a privilege only for those who are already privileged. One has to be born to privilege to enter old age in the first place.

The last NFHS report of 2018 tells us that the life expectancy of Indian women is about 55 years but that life expectancy for Dalit women is about 14 years less (recent figures released by Niti Ayog claim that the average life expectancy of Indian women has now risen to about 70 years but we will have to wait for the next NFHS figures to be released before we can understand the changes that have taken place and also what the caste differentials are.) Meanwhile, a UN study released in 2018 titled *Turning promises into action: gender equality in the 2030 Agenda*, repeats the figures released by the NFHS 4.

Behind these figures are tragic truths. The life expectancy of Indian women is much lower than of women in other societies. Since these figures are average figures, another tragic truth is that women of the non-Dalit communities who are poor and victims of different forms of gender-discrimination, also die young, often in their late forties. As far as Dalit women are concerned, since figures relating to them have been given in the report, a gap of 14 years in their life expectancy is a truly tragic and horrific comment on the poverty, injustice, and sheer exhaustion that they experience.

According to the report, *In India*, a woman aged 20-24 from a poor, rural household is over five times as likely as one from a rich, urban household to marry before the age of 18. There is also an over 20 times likelihood of the former as compared to the latter to have never attended school, 1.3 times not having access to money of her own, and 2.3 times not having a say in spending.

If she is landless and belongs to a scheduled caste, the likelihood of poverty increases, and if she chooses to work, her lack of education and low status in the social hierarchy are likely to result in exploitative working conditions.

The NFHS 4 report, echoes these findings, revealing more tragic truths. In the age-group 25-49, 55.9% Dalit women and 44.1% non-Dalit women suffer from anaemia. The problems of Dalit women leading to their high mortality rate are compounded by the denial of healthcare to them not only because of poverty but because of caste-discrimination. As many as 70% of the women interviewed by the NFHS said that they had faced these problems. 25% of Dalit women and about 17% of non-Dalit women are undernourished. These figures are not only unconscionably high but, once again, bring out the caste-differential.

Of course, poor women, Dalit women, Adivasi women are beautiful, graceful and possessors of great dignity. The tragic truth, however, is that most of them do not live very long, most of them are denied an old age and too many of them grow old at an age that the privileged regard as 'early middle age'.

Growing old in any condition, with or without beauty, grace and dignity is, therefore, linked to caste and class privilege, linked to accidents of birth. Within this cocoon of privilege, who are the women who grow old, beautiful, gracious and dignified without the help of various kinds of implants, surgery and artificial aids? From what I have seen and known, commitment to progressive principles, compassion and a strong sense of service are what have made many women that I have been fortunate to have known grow into old age blessed with all these attributes.

33
AGEING IS MANDATORY.
IT IS A BOON AND A BLESSING.
PADMA SETH

Life is the greatest blessing. A boon to be born as a human being growing from childhood to adolescence, youth, adulthood, and old age. This natural process is mandatory. No one can reverse the process. Bodily growth can be involuntary. But the inner self, which we call "mind", alerts us, and teaches us to be on the right track.

Ageing is also an unavoidable link from the past to present to the future. Memory and imagination are ingrained parts of life. Life is to live and enjoy the numerous possibilities, both positive and negative. In our Indian society we show reverence to ageing and to the aged. But in the West, they think the aged are incompetent and are of no avail to society. It is necessary to understand that age is only a number. Growing up is a choice. It is different from growing old.

It is common knowledge that one is born to grow. Each stage in life brings its own desires and demands. The body-mind combo is a compact reality. The inner energy propels growth of both body and mind. During this growing process, our thinking also changes from time to time. Thus the quality of growth depends on how you utilise the fund of energy from within. Physical growth is programmed while qualitative growth depends on how you feel within: one may respect the inner voice or reject it. One can grow and age even without any understanding of how to take care of one's body and mind.

Early exposure to values in childhood makes us strong. I developed a fascination to be bold and to think freely. As part of growing up in society, we are expected to respect and follow social dictums and age-old practices. In conventional homes our movements and actions are conditioned by faith and beliefs. A widow, a single Brahmin, and a cat are considered bad omens and we are expected to avoid them before moving out of the house. A rebel in me from childhood disbelieved them. I wanted to prove this belief wrong. Wantonly, I would make sure to to meet a widow, a Brahmin or a cat, even any one of them crossing my way. Then alone would I venture to go to school to answer my exams. I always passed with credit. My crusade against superstition continued until I grew old, I could motivate many to shun these abominable beliefs and practices. I hated to see my widowed aunt kept out of auspicious events like marriage and festivities. My mission in life started by openly condemning such practices. Thus I paved for myself a new way of life and a bold journey. I realised, I could be different from my siblings in thought and action. While my sister thought to excel in studies is to set an example for others, I believed in exploring nature, people around, and watch birds, bees and insects. I wanted to fly like Shelly's skylark. Realising that humans are not endowed with flying capabilities, I penned my flying thirst into a poem. Born into a harmonious family of a loving father and mother, we loved peace, joy and laughter. Father taught us to repeat the sentence, "I am Strong, I am Healthy". That autosuggestion turned into a strong belief. Even in old age, this mantra keeps all of us on track. We children could imbibe values of sharing and caring from our gentle parents and grandparents, to empathise and help all in need. All these traits grew stronger day by day up to our old age. We could not see pain in others. Our efforts in counselling others to throw out the feeling of pain or hurt, saved many from huge health complications.

Age Is Only a Number. Who Can Say I Cannot Work When Retired?

Who do we call aged?

- Those who comply with chronological age.
- Those apparently looking aged due to either poor health, or because of sad events that have occurred in their lives.
- Those who are infirm, weak, suffering many ailments in old age.
- Those who have almost lost the zest to live and keep aloof from others and the world at large.
- It is the societal assessment of the person's age, to call them "aged"?

To sum up, it is easy to go by the government or census records, because to put "aged" as a category, the record appears to be the possible parameter to assess the numbers in that age group who have retired from active working life. But this does not detract from their emotional and caring presence, experience, and advice. There is fear that even younger ones may be grouped in such a category if they are negative in their outlook, unproductive in action and are irresponsible, who may appear older than they really are.

When I was told I had reached my age of retirement, I wondered, "How am I aged? All my faculties were in shape, and my zest to continue to work in Bal Bhavan never faded. Soon, thanks to a government project given to me to write on women decision-makers in peace and disarmament, I was kept busy. I never learnt to sit idle. Engaging myself in productive pursuits made me happy. It became difficult for me to accept that I could not be engaged in work simply because I was supposed to be "aged". Age is after all a number. It does not deprive me of my ability or passion to serve. No person or rule can brand me unfit to serve just because I have reached a certain age. Of course, all my productive contributions continue to linger on in my unfading memory. These keep me happy and fulfilled. Having nurtured Bal Bhavan for twelve long years, did not remind me of my age, though an anxiety haunted me with fear and hope that work of Bal Bhavan might not be passed on to wrong hands, after I left. The service rules had called me aged in the records. Why did I refuse to reconcile with this professional interpretation, I truly wondered? Positive attitude is what is important in growing up and in what people call ageing.

All my productive work can easily date when I have been ageing. Registering the Indian Trust for Innovation and Social Change as an NGO in 2000, could train women masons, and auto mechanics. Besides conducting a research project for the Planning Commission on socio-economic conditions leading to maternal and infant mortality in villages, I was able to write a book on the same. This involved visits to six states, 18 districts and 36 villages to collect authentic data. I started womens self-help groups in twelve interior villages in Chhata tehsil in western Uttar Pradesh. I was already aged when I started a Mahila Printing Press in the All India Women's Conference and was able to run a cost effective training programme for 40 girls in compositing and printing. We obtained treadle printing machines free from the Directorate of Printing and the women were kept productively occupied. Also, I could obtain orders for printing of lakhs of labels for the Directorate.

It was truly satisfying to run Balwadis in Ministers' Car garages in Lodi estate, for 4 hours daily, where the children were given free milk. In the process, we could orient their parents about cleanliness and hygiene.

I was a member of the NCW which fully engaged us in work, day and night. It is hard to count the number of cases Mohini Giri, Syeda and I settled through the Parivarik Mahila Lok Adalats which were held even in far away Andaman Nicobar islands. I still remember how the NCW challenged the Chief Justice of Bombay High Court and still managed to rehabilitate the minors retrieved from brothels. Our experience, our knowledge of law and our determination to send the girls to a home mattered. Our ageing was not a disability but a strength. It is amusing to recall that as a result of a telephone talk from Madurai airport with the Chief Minister of Tamil Nadu we obtained a promise of 5 lakhs as compensation for rehabilitating the wrongly-harassed and imprisoned women and children of Ottapadi village. Through this issue we were able to bring public awareness on the plight of 7,000 odd persons who were terrorised by the local Panchayat. We got the village Panchayat President of the same village dismissed and removed from the Dravida Munnetra Kazhagam party. We were old by the government definition, but that did not bar us from putting every ounce of energy to ensure justice for the poor and the weak.

My socially-active life started after retirement. My understanding of issues around became clear and candid. Never once did I remember that I was supposed to retire from active life. How is it possible for anyone else to dictate my action and movements and to decide for me when I am to retire? After all, positive thinking, productive action and good intention and strong determination are needed to bring back natural order in society and in individuals' lives.

It is not a universal truth that all aged are sick and suffer infirmities. I would have fallen sick if I was without work. To keep the body fit, top spiritual gurus and medical professionals do believe positive attitude of mind is necessary. Those who are engaged and prone to complaining and remain normally dissatisfied all the time deserve to be called "negative persons", and not "aged." A youth or an adult all the time gloating over their own needs and image is a bad example to emulate. But "aged" is not to be taken as a bad word. Nor does it denote less activity nor depleting energy levels. Societal and collective pronouncements creating infirm images of the elderly usher wrong signals. Many aged are stronger than those in the prime of their youth. Social conditioning of the aged to keep themselves far away from physical activities and from participating in youthful vocations does trap their freedom of action. This segregation of people in society on the basis of age alone has been proved wrong by energetically aged ones.

Many long years of working in different vocations, gaining the art of public relations, sharing ones work and knowledge, and inter action with colleagues and friends around have left the aged with a lifetime of experience, so they have much to offer by way of knowledge and skills. Classifying people by their age and treating them as outcasts from service have deprived the nations of treasures of knowledge and skills. The pervading illiteracy and ignorance continue due to lack of infrastructure that is costly, plus involving heavy investments needed for engaging young people and professional trainers. It would be pragmatic and cost efficient if we engaged active and positive older people in the education of the young and illiterate.

The Aged, and Their Challenges

Unlike the aged who are fit and healthy, a large number of the aged have to face challenges of body and mind. The process of ageing brings with it issues of failing strength and creeping fears of slowing reflexes, gradual loss of memory, and depleting energy. These may be due to social conditioning and collective expectation of the aged to distance themselves from active life. While enlightened families understand the physical and mental conditions of the aged and their needs, the poor may not be able to cater effectively to their needs. Amongst women in our conventional societies, once the husband dies, it is common to trap the widow within multifold deprivations. The aged widows depend on their families to access even their basic needs. There occurs a lot of suffering by the aged. Besides physical dependency on others, their own perception of their hopelessness emphasises their disabilities. Herein is the need to understand one's inner strength and build up one's own confidence. This can lead to better perception of oneself and of one's energy.

Intention and Determination Are Two Mantras

The aged who are strong can motivate the weak and the frightened, to realise their innate strength, which can help and improve their body and mind. Common social dictums expect them to busy themselves in temples and prayers to God. After all, being human, they carry unquenched desires. Very few others find time or interest to hear their stories. Thus they carry on with suppressed emotions. Loneliness and a feeling of utter neglect by near and dear ones have been the cause for concern for the aged. Such a state of mind leads them to depression. Once they get to live amongst caring people, they feel stronger. Appreciation for their happy disposition brings cheer. What truly makes them alive and happy is engaging them constantly in doing things. Engaging them in conversation individually or in groups improves their persona. While efforts continue at governmental level to design policies to help and rehabilitate the needy, voluntary institutions and individuals with empathy try to bring smiles to their lives. To teach the uncared for is to create an environment where they can feel they are wanted. To come out of their guilt and despair, they get release by offering help to the needy and the vulnerable - for example, orphans who long for affection and attention. Life can be lived under any circumstance by focusing it on a pleasant duty towards the poor and the needy. No scriptures of any faith have segregated the aged, who deserve the highest attention and respect for the many long years of ups and downs of life. Attributing a sense of hopelessness to the aged is unbecoming of a responsible society. Strong intention and unswerving determination are the true mantras to combat the challenges of old age.

Examples to Emulate

An erstwhile Governor of the state of Bihar hit upon an idea to help the aged to feel wanted. This resulted in social restructuring of the children's orphanage and attaching it to the Vanaprastha Ashram of the aged, in Patna. This brought amazing transformation in the lives of the aged who now acted as grandparents of the orphaned children. Thus the campus, filled with utter joy, became an example for many others to copy and emulate. Such cost-effective reforms brought immense, joy and a sense of responsibility to the aged to take care, groom and fill the void in their own lives, as well as tap their potential and to help in the transformation of the children's lives.

At an individual level, the aged cannot lose sight of their immense potential and untapped energy within. The very realisation of this truth can transform them into positive and active human beings.

Mangalam Project

To quote another instance, a village project called Mangalam was initiated by the National Commission of Women (NCW). Former Justice of the Supreme Court Justice Krishna Iyer and Prof. Madhava Menon guided the NCW to choose the smallest state of Puducherry to experiment on how the village women, though illiterate and ignorant, could give justice to themselves. Thirty-odd aged women daily wagers were paid day wages for joining a training workshop. The dishevelled and worn-out looking women had no sense of their own identity except as an unskilled labourer, or an illiterate woman. The trainers simulated situations that required their response. Each one was to tie a black ribbon from their head to bottom to show how totally ignorant they were. When questioned on how to save a corner hut from catching fire, all in chorus shouted that they would call one and all and rush to stop the fire, by pouring sand and water and saving the possessions in the house. When asked why would they do that, the simple reply was, that if their own huts caught fire, there would be no one to help them, so joint-action was essential. The workshop trainers then told then that they clearly had the capacity to take immediate decisions, were aware of the solutions, and they had empathy for others. This was their potential, a veritable treasure for them. The same women then came fully cleaned and dressed up in the evening, looking an intelligent lot after they had realized their own potential. The transformation in them after self realization was amazing. It takes no time to realise one's own strength, you only need awareness of it.

The Aged and Home Remedies

Not all remote areas have hospitals. For simple ailments, people depend on homemade remedies that were passed on from generation to generation. Many homeopaths held medical camps and cured many. This proved less costly than allopathic medicines. Since I watched my Homeo Doctor mother-in-law dispensing free medicines to patients, I learnt about a few ailments and their cure. Amazingly, many thanked me for curing them. I felt elated to find that I could help some cases. The happiness that gave was a lot more than the sense of possessions we own. Life can be sustained with simple treatments, not only by admitting patients to hospital, which is often very costly and a drain on savings.

Positive Thinking and Wellbeing

Feelings of hurt, sadness, and loneliness are also causes of depression. The important lesson that all should realise is that the feeling of guilt within is the cause of deadly diseases, even cancer. Eschewing these unhealthy feelings can bring wonders in ones' health. Positive thinking, forgiving oneself and others for wrong words or deeds also helps to better health. The body sends signals from time to time. Curing oneself is possible at an early stage by attending to the early signals. If overlooked, the negative signals get stronger and vitiate the possibilities of settling the system back to its health stage. In your body and mind interaction, you take instructions from the mind. But in unhappy lives, they are taking instructions from their moods. This causes depression, despair. That means, your intelligence has gone against you. This amply proves how body and mind need to be synchronised to have a healthy system in place. Therefore right feelings are necessary for a strong and healthy body. It is very necessary for the aged to realize how positivity is essential for one's well being.

What is needed for the ageing is to shun self pity, and to stop constant complaining about things and people. To get engaged in physical work turns one's attention to other's needs, which often extends into offering them emotional support. Feeling good under all circumstances is an important mantra for the old. When one's own children have discarded one as a burden on their time and resources, then take the opportunity to discover the world at large, which is eagerly waiting and looking for empathy, love, and affection After all what is life for if not to share and bring joy to the uncared-for and neglected young and old?

Gandhiji said, "Change yourself, and the world around you will change". Age is no bar to help making that change. When you dislike violence on women, widows, the poor, homeless and orphans, you can be bold to condemn and to act against limitations on liberty, equality, and fraternity. Any step towards doing that encourages you to think that you have a role to play. This is how change against wrong thinking and action starts. When you feel strongly against any unhealthy practice in our society, or against any of its numerous superstitions, you muster strength to share your views with others. Once you are convinced that these wrongs need to be rooted out, your strong determination irrespective of your age can think and devise strategies to eliminate them.

Ageing and Challenges; Meticulously Curated for Both Young and Old.

The aged are part and parcel of humanity. They cannot be looked at as an unproductive part of our population. They have a right to lead a comfortable life after serving all their working life. In India, a law exists that stipulates and demands that old parents shall be taken care of by their children, both boys and girls. In case of neglect, the children of the aged parents are liable for due punishment. Legally, it is the bounden duty of the sons and daughters to take care of the old parents who nurtured them, kept them away from worries and protected them from harm. Emotional support is equally essential as economic or financial care of the aged parents. This is a natural way how societies maintain gratitude, harmony and peace amongst young and old within the family, the society and the country as a whole.

In spite of what has been said, ageing people face numerous challenges including psychological symptoms of uncertainties in behaviour. Mental health is equally important for the aged. Depression, anxiety lead to dementia. To keep cognitive fitness of the aged is important. Suppressed emotions have to be brought out. Ups and downs in life are unavoidable. It all depends on how you turn it into Positive thinking. The capacity to change your perception is what matters. In order to keep the mind energetic the body needs to be engaged in continuous activities of doing something useful for all. Living in congenial surroundings, or living with individuals or groups in similar circumstances are important to imbibe learning, work, activity and behaviour.

Science has opened up minds to think beyond boundaries. Technology has transformed life. It can stall the process of ageing by modern techniques of transplanting the affected organs of the body. Technology is gradually replacing the need for memory and imagination. When with press of a button, one is getting answers to every question and query, artificial intelligence is slowly introducing robotic characteristics in human beings that are pushing human yearning for speeding up time and action. Researches in greater numbers are diminishing the valued legacy of the aged.

But there is another aspect to ageing in today's times. The vast majority of the ageing are poor. The young ones are almost discarding the old as problematic and a drain on their time and resources. Most of the rich sons and daughters prefer to leave their old parents in posh old age homes unmindful of the monthly or yearly fees they have to pay. Hitherto meticulously curated interdependence and inter exchange of emotions in relationships in families, have kept societies as self supporting and happy. Today due to self-centred social ethics, the aged have lost the reverence and respect that was part of the Indian cultural ethos..

The mechanical and technical intelligence are eroding the natural human faculties and skills. . The new war has begun between technology and the greatest asset of humanity, which is human intelligence. It will not be out of place to reiterate that the aged are natural and spontaneous feeders and inculcators of human values and concerns, and sustainers of emotional bonding between the very young and the old. The aged and the ageing have the onus of bridging the increasing gulf between the very young and the old.

I Am a Proud Aged Person. I Assert My Inner Strength and Energy, Eschew Self Pity, Do not Complain, and Find Satisfaction in Action.

I am proud to announce that I am the most lived and living Senior Citizen called the aged. Even during the Lockdown in almost eight months, I have been able to keep busy counselling the ones who sought help and could retrieve a girl abducted with the help of the Police.

Finally my mantra for positive ageing is:

- Believe in self help, but make it a point to thank all those who care for you and help you in need.
- Do not indulge in self pity and hating people, Discard jealousy, pettiness, complaining and crying. These are negative emotions. Positive thinking is not only for your own wellbeing but it helps all those around you. When you are peaceful, you enjoy being alive.
- Do not lose sight of your immense potential and the untapped inner energy,
- Do remember that our life on Earth is to live and make others happy, Kindness breeds love and affection
- Remove small hurt and pain. The sooner you get them out of the system, the better you feel.
- Do not hoard things for your own use. Share what you possess, your skills, your fund of experience. Find happiness in giving and sharing. Once you share, you are no less than a caregiver.

- Constantly appreciating what life has offered and be thankful to feel good.
- "I am Strong. I am healthy". By such utterances, one gets rejuvenated and is able to extend oneself to others and to remain happy and cheerful. When you are exuberant within, problems will turn into possibilities and life will not look burdensome and long.

34
MANTRAS FOR GROWING OLD GRACEFULLY
DR. URMIL SHARMA

A young woman is a gift of nature; an old woman is a work of art. But growing old gracefully and elegantly is a progression that is in your hands.

What is in our hands is to follow healthy steps to grow old gracefully and glowingly.

Prayer:- Prayer brings the mind into purity and tranquillity. Prayers undo all the knots of our worries. Prayer results in faith, and faith is the highest form of conviction, positive energy and increased courage. As medicines help in curing a disease, prayer purifies a sick soul. I have found the Gayatri Mantra as a very effective prayer as it is an invocation to the life giving and life sustaining energy of the Sun- energy which sustains all ages of humanity

Gayatri Mantra:- O God! The giver of life. Remover of pains and sorrows, Bestower of happiness and joy. Creator of the universe. We meditate on Thee. May Thou inspire and guide our intellect in the right direction.

Happiness:- is indeed the best cosmetic, radiates you with joy and peace within us which is covered by ignorance: one has to tap it to discover it oneself.

Meditation:- is an important tool and key to open every pore of the body, mind and soul to peace, happiness and contentment. It opens fountains of the spiritual power. Meditation makes us realize that we are all actually lovable, peaceful souls and that our true nature is to appreciate and love everyone, connecting our souls in an ocean of peace. We become powerful and speak the truth, overcome ego, anger, jealously, hatred, revenge, greed, fear, back-biting, negative thoughts; and we see only good qualities in an individual and ignore negative ones.

Some pointers to ageing gracefully:

- Selfishness leads to self destruction
- Faith is your banner
- Courage is first virtue
- Compassion is the best virtue
- Love is the highest virtue. Love rules without the sword and binds with a chord.
- Truth is that virtue by possessing which all virtues cling to you.
- Accept everyone as they are.
- No grudge to be held. Hoarding old grudges in the mind deprives you of positive energy, and negative energy radiates to the body.
- Emotional ill health has to be treated like a disease and cured. Positive emotions energize the body.
- Try to realize your inner potential. It is in your power to be in control of situations

The above were my mantras for the mind that needs to age gracefully. But a healthy mind has to be supported by a healthy body. Certain important foods and herbs act as antibiotic, antiseptic anti-oxidant, detox foods and are anti-cancerous.

Tulsi (Basil): Anti-cancerous; plant that secretes oxygen and purifies the atmosphere continuously, insect repellent. Good digestive; anti-oxidant. Fights stress; excellent with honey.

Haldi (Turmeric): (especially in the raw form) natural steroid, anti-cancerous (especially cancer of the kidney), fights allergy and joint pains.

Amla (Gooseberry): Qualities of mother and nurse, rejuvenates the blood, heart, lungs, joint pains and mouth ulcers.

Lasun (Garlic): anti-cancerous, wonder drug, anti oxidant, antiviral, fights allergy and reduces cholesterol.

Neem/Curry leaves (Azadirachta Indica): anti-cancerous, good for BP & diabetes, anti-viral.

Dalchini (Cinnamon): anti-cancerous, antiseptic, reduces cholesterol, good for heart and digestion.

Aloe vera: excellent for health, makes your face glow and wrinkle free, massage good for migraine, good for hair.

Jeera (Cumin seed): anti-cancerous, good digestive.

Laung (Cloves): anti-bacteria, antiviral, anti fungal.

Adrak (Ginger): blood purifier, antiseptic, anti-infective.

Pyaz (Onion): antioxidant, rich in protein, calcium and iron

Pudina (Mint)/ Menthol: sinuses cure

Important fruits which can combat cancer: grapes, apples, pomegranates, oranges, prunes, grapefruit, mango, peach, strawberry, blueberry, cherries, apricot.

Important vegetables which can hep prevent or even combat cancer: soya, wheatgrass mushrooms, spirulina, olives, lemon.

With positive energy radiating in the body, with a body that has aged but not deteriorated, one can prove that age is just a number.

35
THE BEST IS YET TO BE! GROW OLD ALONG WITH ME
LALITA RAMDAS

"Do not go where the pathways lead –
but go where there are no pathways and leave a trail".

Dancing on a tightrope while juggling half a dozen balls in the air .... My favourite image of myself!

When I received a message from Mohini Giri and the Guild of Service a few days ago – asking me to share some thoughts and reflections about my personal experience of growing older, "so very gracefully"as she sweetly and tactfully put it, my instinctive response was a yes, and also that I would get it done by the deadline.

At that time, I did not factor in a totally unscheduled second cyclonic storm which hit us in the Alibag area of the Konkan coast in spurts over three days.

For those who have not had the experience of living in a rural area with minimal and ageing infrastructure, this meant battening down all objects which might potentially fly around because of the unpredictable high velocity of winds – not to mention finding ways of keeping heavy rains out and worrying about all the damage to recently-planted vegetables and all the paddy which was almost ready for harvesting.

Along with the rest of the physical infrastructure, our own physical and mental infrastructure are also under stress. Like many millions across our land, we have been learning to be more stoic, resign ourselves to endure what cannot be cured, and smile through it all.

So, over the past week we have been hearing the same refrain – our fields are water logged and the *dhaan* has fallen and completely submerged. So, as they dig gullies to drain out the water, we are all anxiously watching the skies and praying that the ominous clouds will move on and drop their load elsewhere!

We had also watched the skies in June, with hope and expectation of rain, so that paddy could be planted. And then boom!! Nisarga came, the first cyclone to hit the west coast in a century, that laid low our district. But for the first time we are also hearing whispered rumours of the jobless, no food, and seeing no alternative to taking their own lives. This is our rural reality, in spite of the fact that we live in a relatively well to do region.

The Shift to Bhaimala – A Village in the Konkan

Twenty-six years ago, in a completely unplanned set of events, Ramu and I found ourselves driving in an Armada van, packed from floor to top of the roof top carrier, with basic minimum requirements to run a home and kitchen, an old tent, and our faithful companion, Spitok the Big Black Lab who had journeyed from the luxury of many navy houses to this relatively wild and vast rural area. So one may well ask the question, "Why did you, at the ages respectively of sixty and offifty-three, decide to ride out like young pioneers into the wild west so to speak, when most people would have happily settled for a comfortable suburban retirement life style?"

After a lifetime spent in the secure embrace and ambience provided by the armed forces, and the confidence that one's *roti*, *kapda* and some form of *makaan* would always be guaranteed; and despite the disruptions of endless transfers, new places, people, schools and cultures, for the most part represented a way of existence which presented no real threats or challenges. We certainly were among the privileged who led highly protected existences which immunises us to the reality faced by over 70% of our people. Growing up in a typical middle-class household, with a mix of progressive and traditional norms imparted by my parents, it was the nuns and teachers of the convent where I studied who primarily shaped my persona, my ideas and personality, conforming, non-argumentative and well behaved!

And some decades later it was another nun and priest who knocked the hell out of all my years of convent socialisation.... And like a phoenix I rose from the ashes of my old self in a form totally unanticipated!

The move to this seven-acre piece of barren land in a small village in Alibag *taluka* was both unplanned and unexpected. The land itself was granted by the Government of Maharashtra to Ramu for his gallantry award of a Vir Chakra in the 1971 war. And this has shaped our actions and provided us challenges, opportunities and insights that could never have happened had we continued in suburbia. The symbiotic affinity to the land even led to our being caught up in a long battle to fight to save 22 villages, including ours. The 22 Gaon Bachao Andolan has secured its place in local history annals by struggling for four years against a predatory take-over attempt by Government together with a private real estate developer under the infamous Special Economic Zone scheme. We never imagined that we would see my husband, a former service chief, leading a *Rasta Roko* or giving a speech from atop a jeep right in front of the Collectorate!

Love, Marriage, Children – A Typical Pattern?

Falling in love at the age of 21, with the man with whom I have now lived for 59 years, and deciding to follow my heart rather than pursue the opportunity to study in the USA, was a big decision. Having three children in quick succession, dealing with a series of their major congenital health issues, and yes, being a 'dutiful' mother and naval wife, more or less determined my own trajectory up to my mid thirties. For sure, I did not rock any boats, except a few domestic ones. Many influences and events helped to build my trajectory. But as with all of us, there are some events which stand out and become powerful determinants of future directions. And the best I can do in the course of this limited account is to highlight a few which I count as significant because they impacted many of my decisions and priorities.

Education for Subversion or Domestication

As the ferment of questioning and rebelliousness within me was growing, I guess it was only inevitable that in 1977, while teaching in St Anne's School in Mumbai, I was among a bunch of teachers who signed up for a workshop titled "Education to Reality". And what an education it turned out to be, mind blowing in its impact! Personally, for me, this intensive structural analysis of our economic, political, social, cultural and religious system and structure, was like a ruthless stripping away and stripping down of everything I had hitherto thought and believed to be true. It also strongly drove home the point that the root causes could be traced back to our education system which had domesticated our minds, and conditioned us to accept rather than question, challenge or debate. Lord Macaulay had succeeded beyond all belief. This innocuous 'workshop' marked the stirrings of my 'political' awakening and my life has not been the same since! My avatar as a naval wife who was largely unquestioning, had suddenly undergone a radical transformation – and I metamorphosed into what today we subsume under that all embracing word, "activist".

The process of peeling away the layers of the onion right down to its core, so to speak, was both painful and traumatic. It was ironic that what one set of nuns had carefully crafted over many years through what was a much sought after "schooling" had been ruthlessly dismantled by another nun and priest! Gabe and Gladys were well schooled in Liberation Theology, which led to an interesting cross-fertilisation of several streams of ideology, philosophy and faith systems. "Education to Reality" held up a mirror to our education system and exposed how it had deliberately kept us distanced from and blind to, the harsh political, economic and social realities and oppressive structures of our country and our people. Liberation theology spread rapidly across many countries and sectors. The idea that conscientisation and de-schooling as conceptualised by thinkers like Paolo Freire, could become a powerful tool to encourage young minds to question, think and reflect on everything they heard, read and experienced around them, was stimulating. It also raised hopes in many of us who wanted to see a much greater degree of churning after the experience of the Emergency in India, that this should lead to a rigorous process of questioning and independent action, which would become the basis for a stronger and healthier democracy. The ideas were intoxicating and the potential for positive change was seemingly endless.

Multiple Churnings – Internal Rumblings

But the subversive ideas also created a prolonged period of turbulence within my family! With their mother turning into an activist from the traditional mom who was always there to open the front door and greet them on their return from school with brownies and hot snacks, this created resentment, anxiety and outright hostility at times in the minds of our girls. As far as the spouse was concerned, for him it meant dealing with a newly charged, more argumentative and different persona altogether. This also meant a wife who was now less amenable to sparing time to be available for cocktail parties and coffee mornings as was often expected of us service wives. In 1978, we moved to Delhi – our first posting at Naval Head Quarters. And I was a very different Me. The family continued to have long and sometimes not so friendly discussions. "Why is this so important? What's the point? Why can't you be like other mothers? You are now always running off to some *basti*, some meeting or some rally or *juloos*?' While I was excited and so wrapped up in my new-found causes, for those around me it was a tough struggle to figure out what was going on.

I was scarcely to be found at home. There was always a burning issue, a march to the boat club, a *dharna* at Ram Lila grounds. Even when there were official events, like a banquet at the Rashtrapati Bhavan, i would arrive home barely in time to do a quick change, not particularly bothered about whether blouse and sari matched the accessories, but more concerned that sheets of questionnaires and petitions were carefully stuffed into my evening bag, so that I could solicit signatures from the VIPs present!

How we survived those early rocky days of my activist role is still hard to believe. Most other husbands would have told someone like me to "shape up orship out". And my family and friends said openly to me that they did not recognise me any more. But this really speaks volumes for my husband, Ramu, a remarkable and open-minded human being like few others, and luckily our relationship withstood this most severe test and our marriage has survived 59 years which even as I write, we celebrate today.

Laying the Foundations of the Many Peoples' Movements

It was a time like no other, and the years between 1978 and 1987 saw one of the most intensive periods I have known. Long term relationships and friendships were made and cemented during this time, and they continue till today, both individual and organisational, covering everything from human rights to women's rights, ecology and environment, National Literacy Mission, anti-communal and anti-nuclear work to name a few. Street theatres on dowry and rape, the Mathura Rape case, the deepening circles of understanding about sexual violence and the roots of patriarchy, holding public meetings and discussions and taking street plays out into *mohallas* and residential colonies and universities. And even as we criticised the government of the day, the political parties, and made our voices heard loud and clear, we also were fully aware of the great gift of our democracy and the Constitution. We were indeed grateful to both since it gave us the freedom to criticise and exercise the right to dissent.

In the early eighties a group of us believing in the power of education and the need for a liberating model, came together to set up ANKUR – Society for Alternatives in Education. Ankur continues today some three decades down the line – growing from strength to strength. As much as I was totally committed to my new found calling of political and community activism, I was also committed to being a caring and supportive partner to my husband who was climbing the ladder to higher command positions. In 1983, Ramu was appointed to command the Eastern Fleet base in Vishakapatnam. Since our girls were at critical board exam stages, I stayed on in Delhi, and it was thus that I found myself caught up in the events leading up to and the aftermath of the 1984 tragedy in Delhi.

The assassination of PM Indira Gandhi and the genocidal violence that followed was another watershed moment, a defining line where the naïve trust in the 'benign' nature of the state was finally abandoned. Large numbers of us (citizens, students, academics, housewives and others) threw ourselves into relief, rehabilitation, interventions, documentation. Personally, I was co-ordinating a relief camp at Nanaksar, and it was interesting that a large number of the young people who worked with me then have been among those active handling the fallout from a range of subsequent communal disturbances, including the most recent protests in Delhi against Citizenship Amendment Act 2019. For almost three years, a group of us from civil society groups worked with the survivors, moved with them from the camps to their resettlement locations, and understood, from inside, the long term impact on the destruction of trust and the resultant wounded psyches. It was an important eye opener for me and many other women who are torn between duty, commitment, and conscience. I was advised by many well-meaning colleagues NOT to get involved in the process of reports and testifying before Enquiry Commissions constituted to look into the 1984 Pogrom [I refuse to call them Riots] – because it would affect my husband's career and promotions.

With all the constraints of the existing communication system, somehow Ramu and I were able to speak and discuss this. The bottom line was this: "Follow your conscience, don't worry about my career. You have worked night and day and I know the intensity of your feelings. Feel free to go ahead and testify". And I did. Lessons are never learned from history – 1984, 1992 – Babri Masjid, and the Bombay blasts, and then 2002. And the battle for the idea and the soul of India had already been joined.

In what was still the future, this was to lead me and Ramu too into a decade-long engagement and involvement with the Movement for Nuclear Disarmament and Peace (CNDP), with ongoing actions and campaigns to build People to People Contact with Pakistan and also our neighbours in South Asia through groups like Pakistan India Peoples' Forum for Peace and Democracy (PIPFPD) and IPSI (India Pakistan Soldiers Initiative for Peace).

In 1994, I was elected President of the International Council for Adult Education – a post I held for 5 years and which took me to many countries – learning so much along the way. I was a founder member of Greenpeace India in the late nineties – then became Board Chair – and went on to hold office for four years as the Chair of Greenpeace International.

Meanwhile, back to the late eighties and the balancing act between following our different pathways. I had to move out of Delhi, to accompany Ramu in his two important commands in Kochi and Vishakapatnam. Each of these presented both challenges and opportunities and there is a separate story to tell. I was able to bring into the otherwise very traditional welfarist world of the navy wives, a subtle but important shift to addressing gender and patriarchy, and the familiar issue of violence against women. Thus, I succeeded in creating a network to address disability across the service, and a series of other measures by which the community gradually assumed responsibility for extending a helping hand to children of domestic workers. We built a wider awareness about environment and ecology, and also about education itself. International Women's Day, probably never heard about within navy circles, became an established part of the naval and Navy Wives Calendar by the time we retired in 1993.

I am mentioning this by way of illustration of how being in certain positions of authority and power, by virtue of the posts held by the spouse, can provide opportunities to push for constructive change, as long as one is clear about one's position, does not abuse power, and takes people in the system along. It was a combination of all of these which eventually resulted in the production of the first Gender Sensitisation Module by the navy – to prepare officers and sailors for the induction of women into the armed forces in 1992. The navy was the first of our armed forces to do so. To my delight, the module for sailors and officers, in English and in Hindi, still serves to put personnel through a detailed syllabus and plentiful simulation and other exercises on the readjustment and mind-set change required as more and more women come in to serve in the armed forces.

The Personal Is the Political

This familiar and almost clichéd slogan of the women's movement has resonated deeply with me, and this is lesson number two, as I look back on what I have learned by my years in public life. Don't fear – follow your conscience

Our daughter went to study in the USA, and met a fellow student originally from Pakistan. They fell in love, kept waiting to marry till her naval father retired. But eventually, in 1990, we told them to go ahead, knowing that this might mean being excluded from consideration for the top post in the navy. He informed both the Defence Minister and the then Prime Minister. Both gave their blessings to go ahead and attend the wedding in Chicago. To our pleasant surprise, the Government of India selected Admiral Ramdas to head the Indian Navy from 1990 to 1993. The message is very simply to follow your conscience and to be truthful –in our case, there was no negative consequence.

And finally – a personal talisman for energy and motivation has been to continue to retain a sense of curiosity and excitement, identify and prioritise some goals and issues, and go ahead with doing what excites, angers, and energises you. Be an active citizen and follow the Constitutional dharma. You cannot go wrong.

Today we are 80 and 87 respectively, and yes we are blessed indeed to still have each other as pillars of mutual support. There have been countless amazing role models, some of the most inspiring have certainly been women like Mohini Giri. God bless her.

36

THE ART AND SCIENCE OF AGEING GRACEFULLY

ASHOK SAJJANHAR

Ageing is mandatory. It is a democratic phenomenon. Everyone has to experience it. But like happiness, ageing gracefully is a choice. To a few it comes more naturally and spontaneously than it does to others. Most of us aspire to it and need to work towards achieving it. The more one practises it, the easier it becomes. It can be built like a habit, which becomes second nature with repetition and reiteration.

I don't wish to get into the debate on what defines old age. Is it 65 or 70 or beyond? My own experience tells me that it varies with the individual. I have seen people who are 95 years of age and who still walk ramrod straight, are in full control of their faculties and don't suffer from any major physical or emotional ailments. There are several others who are comparatively much younger but whose spiritual, emotional and physical strength are at a considerably lower level. It is of course quite clear that with the advances in technology and medicine, and with much greater focus on disciplined eating and active living, people are leading lives that are much healthier and also living much longer. It is justly said that today's 60 years is equivalent to 40 years of a few decades ago!

My comments below are borne out of personal experience. Hence they are particularly targeted at the age bracket 60 years and above, because that is the age at which the Government of India stipulates that an individual has transformed into a senior citizen; although it is my strong conviction that in India today, as in many other countries, people can contribute meaningfully to society and nation building for years and decades beyond the age of superannuation.

I have observed that in most cases, as individuals approach this D-Day of completing 60 years and retiring from government, private or public sector enterprises, a pall of gloom descends upon them. There is an impression that this is the end of the world for them, that their standing and prestige in their own eyes and that of their families and society will suffer a huge loss as all their power and authority will be taken away. This impression exists because these people have so intimately identified themselves with what they have been engaged in for so many years that they find it difficult to visualise an existence beyond their offices and usual routines. I have seen many people succumb to such thoughts, thinking themselves worthless and unfit to engage in anything meaningful for themselves or the world at large.

On superannuating from a job or a service, it is my belief that we should immediately distance ourselves from the official position that we were holding and the work we were doing. It is necessary to rediscover and reinvent ourselves. We need to move with the flow of time and circumstances and evolve along with them – allowing ourselves to grow, rather than pining for the past.

In the humdrum of official life and existence there are several things that we might have wanted to do but were not able to find the time for. Some of us who are musically inclined might have been interested in learning vocal music or playing an instrument, or simply listening to music more by attending concerts and performances. Some people might have a latent passion for gardening. Or travelling, or reading, or writing, or painting. They might not have had the time or possibility to pursue these interests during work life. The time following entry into senior citizenhood may be gainfully utilised by engaging in activities that we always fancied but did not get the time to indulge in.

We always need to be open to new opportunities that might sometimes arise out of nowhere. It is not judicious to be too fixated in one's ideas about what we can or should do. We should be ready to accept new challenges. But of course, after having accepted them, we should put in our best effort to ensure that we succeed. We should not limit ourselves to areas in which we have worked our whole lives, but should be willing to explore new pastures as they appear.

To share my own experience, soon after my return from Stockholm on retirement, the opportunity to head the National Foundation for Communal Harmony appeared in a most unexpected manner. I decided to take up the challenge even though before that, I had never engaged directly in the area of domestic policy formulation and implementation. This was particularly so in the sensitive domain of inter-faith amity and tranquillity. It was an amazingly enriching experience that exposed me to a multitude of individuals and organisations that I would otherwise never have come in contact with. Soon after that, by a quirk of chance, I received an opportunity to appear in panel discussions on some national TV channels. Initially I was a little hesitant, but gradually warmed up to the idea. Today, I find it to be an excellent platform to keep myself up to date with the latest developments in global events and Indian foreign policy, while also being in active contact with major thought leaders in these areas.

The most important way to get out of this feeling of depression, which has the potential of becoming a vicious downward spiral, is to re-invent ourselves and consider how our expertise, knowledge and experience can contribute to solving problems that the country and the world are facing. All of us, in our many professions, have had exposure to various challenges. All of this knowledge and skill can be channelled to provide solutions for problems confronted by our proximate societies. It is important to keep in mind that while sharing our know-how and understanding of issues, personal benefit or status should not be a part of the consideration. This is our time to give back to society that which we have been fortunate enough to receive. One way to do this is by sharing our competence with NGOs or similar civil society organisations. We can add immensely to our own happiness and well-being by using our strengths to help those who belong to the impoverished segment of our society. However, if our competence is to be utilised in a commercial venture, there should be no hesitation in accepting a suitable remuneration.

It is necessary to reconcile with the fact that as we get along in years, the spotlight will be taken off us and focused on those who are younger, more active and more powerful in the authority they wield. This is, of course, not valid for artistes, performers, academics and those in public life who "never age" and who, like wine, get better with the passage of time. Some of the most outstanding examples of individuals who have continued to blossom with the flow of years are Dr. Karan Singh, Dr. Mohini Giri, Ambassador Maharaja Krishna Rasgotra, Dr. Kapila Vatsyayan (who sadly passed away recently), Ambassador SK Lambah, Dr. Saroja Vaidyanathan, Dr. Achala Moulik (IAS, eminent author), Dr. Shovana Narayan, Ambassador Pascal Alan Nazareth, Dr. Kalyani Roy (Educationist, and Chairperson of the Cambridge Group of Schools) and several more. All of them have excelled in their chosen fields and have contributed immensely to bringing happiness, knowledge and wisdom to people, making this world a better place.

In addition to dealing with the outside world in a mutually beneficial and satisfying manner, it is equally if not more essential to look inwards and ensure that we are at peace with ourselves and the environment in which we live. As we start getting along in years, it is time to find happiness and satisfaction from within and not from outside. This is something that we need to observe throughout our lives, but as we are so regularly engaged with official work and duties, it becomes difficult to spend adequate quality time with ourselves in the way that we should be doing. In advanced years, this becomes a necessity. Happiness from outward sources is temporary and fleeting. Happiness that comes from within is sustainable and stays with us for a long time. This can be further promoted through cultivating a regular practice of meditation which can help us to be at peace with ourselves.

Some other principles which I have found to be extremely helpful in my day to day life throughout, but particularly over the last few years, are as follows:

The 90-10 Principle: This has been enunciated by the well-known management expert Dr. Stephen Covey. His assertion is that we have no control over 10% of the things that happen to us, but we have full control over the 90% which comprises how we respond to any given situation or development. This 90% determines the happiness in our lives. It's all about how one reacts to situations that occur everyday in our lives. This is as relevant and valuable when we are in the prime of our life, but I find that its significance is greater in advancing years. With the benefit of years and experience, we realise that the significance of any situation is temporary and is not worth spoiling relations with our family or friends or to let the sour taste of an unpleasant happening continue for a long time.

Attitude of Gratitude: This is an extremely powerful tool to maintain balance and peace of mind. It becomes particularly essential during our ageing years. There is a preponderant tendency amongst a majority of people to complain about what they perceive they don't have, while forgetting to be appreciative or mindful of all the blessings that life has showered upon them. I am convinced that an Attitude of Gratitude needs to be cultivated amongst all of us on a constant basis. I suggest that the first thing we should do as we get up in the morning and the last thing before going to bed is to remember a few things that we have to be grateful for and thank the Almighty, irrespective of which faith or religion we belong to, for all that has been bestowed upon us.

Be Positive. Be Optimistic: There can be no greater reward or sense of fulfilment than being happy ourselves and making others happy. If we wish to achieve that pinnacle, the easiest and surest way is to develop a healthy attitude and a positive frame of mind. People tend to find fault with their lives for the most inconsequential things. They unnecessarily worry and make themselves anxious and unhappy by imagining the worst-case scenarios which most of the time never occur. On the other hand, being optimistic and positive imbues one with the energy and enthusiasm to accomplish the task at hand quickly and successfully. This spirit of positivity is particularly required in the twilight years. In addition to the challenges that are required to be confronted due to Covid-19 and the declining economy and worsening pollution, old people have to contend with myriad pains in their bodies and uncertain health conditions.

Be Compassionate. Be Kind: It is essential to be generous, benevolent and sympathetic to those who are not as privileged as we might be. There is a great deal of strife and misery in the world. This has been further compounded by the coronavirus pandemic resulting in huge job losses and health challenges, particularly for the poorer sections of our society. As responsible members of the society and the global community, it is incumbent upon us to do our part to ameliorate the hardships being experienced by our less-fortunate sisters and brethren. Charity can begin at home – we could start by being more generous in taking care of the needs of our personal staff like our domestic helps, drivers, security guards, gardeners etc. There is a special joy in giving which transcends all other forms of happiness. Giving generously is the surest way of increasing the sum total of happiness in the world.

Be Healthy – Do Yoga and Meditate: If we wish to contribute meaningfully and substantially to the world around us, it is imperative that we stay healthy and active. This has several components, but the most important is to eat moderately while ensuring a balanced diet. As Gandhi ji said, one should Eat to Live and Not Live to Eat. This is not to suggest that one should eat frugally and only bland and tasteless food, but it is important to ensure that we eat the right type and in appropriate quantities. As we get along in years, our metabolisms start weakening. It becomes advisable to eat foods that can be digested easily. We should put greater emphasis on vegetables, fruits, nuts and fluids. And to the extent possible, try to avoid red meat, fried food, sugars and alcoholic beverages.

Another important element is to stay active and exercise regularly. There is a tendency to put on unneeded fat because of our sedentary lifestyles as we get along in years. This needs to be avoided by regularly engaging in games and exercises. With the passage of years, strenuous games like tennis and squash need to be avoided, and those who have the possibility should engage themselves with golf or undertaking long treks whenever possible. Regular walks in the mornings and evenings are immensely beneficial but they need to be supplemented with exercise to convert the unwanted fat to muscles. In old age, people tend to accumulate fat at the expense of muscles. This decay of muscles can be highly debilitating when we get into our late70s and 80s. It is essential to build a healthy diet and exercise routine to ensure that we are not confronted with a fait accompli when no remedial action is possible.

Possibly the most beneficial and therapeutic activities for physical as well as mental, emotional and spiritual solace that I have engaged in are yoga, pranayama and meditation. Much has been written on this and spoken about it so I will not delve into this issue in detail except to reaffirm that yoga and meditation restore a balance in our physical and spiritual lives that help us not only deal effectively with the challenges that life throws at us, but also maintain the peaceful and tranquil disposition in the face of myriad obstacles that we might have to contend with. Yoga and meditation are religion-neutral and are used by millions around the world to live better lives.

Keep Yourself Engaged Meaningfully: It is absolutely essential to keep ourselves busy with pursuits that we enjoy and that are also beneficial to the society, our community, our country and the world beyond. If we don't immerse ourselves in things we enjoy doing, we will be forced to unnecessarily focus on issues that do not need or deserve our attention and will result only in creating tension in our minds. And this is possibly the worst mental state to be in, as it will also have psychosomatic repercussions on our health. So, keeping ourselves busy with our hobbies and interests is of enormous importance.

Spend More Time with Family and Friends: Covid 19 has provided a unique opportunity to everyone to connect and spend quality time with their families. This can be the best and biggest source of contentment and relaxation for all of us. In the final analysis, it is close family and a select group of friends that really matter. So rather than expanding our Rolodexes (or Twitter followers) with acquaintances and contacts, it would be much more meaningful to strengthen our bonds with family and close friends.

Get Off the Social Media: I would strongly suggest that senior citizens avoid venturing onto social media platforms like Twitter which can be divisive and toxic. These can have the unintended consequence of raising anxiety levels which can be particularly harmful for senior citizens.

Stop Watching News Channels: Instead, Watch Netflix: On a slightly lighter note, I would like to suggest that to the extent possible, senior citizens need to avoid watching private Indian news channels which often force those who are watching them to descend into depths of gloom and despair. Instead there are several gentle, soft, inspiring and motivational serials on Netflix and other OTT platforms which can be both uplifting and instructive and relaxing.

Identify Role Models: I am sure that all of us know some people who put into practice all that has been mentioned above. Such people need not necessarily be from the field or area that we are pursuing but their determination, commitment and single-minded devotion inspires everyone to make the best use of their time in advancing years. I could give a sterling example in my own immediate family of my father-in-law Shri Rabindra Kapur. He is over 90 years old. He retired from a senior government position more than 3 decades ago. He has kept himself very agile and active, physically and professionally, and has been at the forefront of helping others. My mother in law sadly passed away a few years ago, and he found himself at a loose end. But he did not allow fate to determine his state of mind and health. He was always keen to learn to play the flute, but during all these years, he never got the time to devote himself to that pursuit. So, after the unfortunate demise of his wife, he started taking lessons to play the flute at the Triveni Kala Sangam in New Delhi. He would go there three times every week to attend these classes. These have come to a temporary stop over the last six months because of Covid, but he uses this time to practice at home what he has learnt at Triveni. In addition, being a keen swimmer, he goes regularly to his club for his morning swim. He is also a yoga enthusiast and does more than an hour of yoga practice every day. Till a few months ago, he would take his dog out for morning and evening walks and drive himself to nearby places. Being healthy, active and energised is part of his identity. In his own understated and modest way, he sets an example for all who come in contact with him, that with the right attitude, habits and discipline, we can handle all the adversities that life throws our way.

It is said that age is just a number. To make it truly so, it is essential to prepare ourselves suitably. I have done my best to use all of the above *mantras* to navigate through the journey of life. One of my favourite quotes that I have often shared with my children is as follows –"May God grant me the Courage to change the things I can; Serenity to accept the things I cannot, and Wisdom to know the difference." At this time in life, we must leverage the wisdom that we have accumulated over the years to accept many things that have changed, but also find the courage to act on what is in our control. Find the courage to reinvent ourselves, to explore new sides to ourselves, and also to invest in positive, healthy habits for our minds and bodies.

It might seem difficult at first, but it is certainly possible. The benefits are well worth the effort that we put in for ourselves, for our immediate families and friends, and for the world at large.

I wish all readers of this article, senior citizens or otherwise, good health, happiness, peace of mind and contentment in their lives.

37

THE ART OF AGEING POSITIVELY, PRODUCTIVELY AND GRACEFULLY

ARUN BHARAT RAM

I want to start by congratulating the Guild for completing 50 glorious years of service to our great nation. Over the years, the Guild has been able to make a very meaningful and sustainable impact on the lives of vulnerable people in their quest to gain a voice in India's social and economic discourse. I want to especially congratulate Mohini ji for her leadership of this great institution. My wife, Manju and I have been privileged to have had the opportunity to support the activities of the Guild. In fact, Manju and I were living in Madras (now Chennai), India, when she joined the Guild for Service in the city and became an active member until we returned to Delhi in 1981. Manju was approached by Mohini ji to continue her work with the Guild in Delhi, which she did with total commitment. My introduction to Mohini ji was also through Manju, who was by then deeply involved with the Guild.

I am happy to learn that on the 50th anniversary of the Guild, you are planning to bring out a publication on the Art of Ageing – positively, productively and gracefully.

I ran Shri Ram Fibres, a company I founded along with my father, Dr. Bharat Ram in 1970 for more than 40 years. Since Shri Ram Fibres's incorporation in 1970 and the subsequent establishment of our first plant in Manali, near Chennai, India in 1974, we have seen it grow from being a single unit tyre cord manufacturer into a leading, diversified chemical conglomerate today. I am very proud of what we have been able to achieve at Shri Ram Fibres (SRF).

The satisfaction that one gets when one is able to build a vibrant, value-based and innovative organization is unparalleled. An organization that has the capability to meet the challenges and aspirations of our future generation is extremely fulfilling. At the same time, it is very important for any leader to ensure a smooth transition to the next generation of leaders, who can fulfil their own dreams and ambitions, while keeping the ethos and the core values of the organization intact.

No matter how good things are, I believe that there is always scope to make it even better. Pursuing our passion for continuous improvement, we try to seize each moment as an opportunity to create greater value.

That has been our unrelenting commitment at SRF.

Since my retirement from active day-to-day management of the company about fifteen years ago, I have lived my life pursuing different goals and interests, as time went along. During this period, my wife was with me. We were avid theatre goers, travellers and art collectors. In fact, Manju and I went on long holidays and travelled to many countries that we had not visited in the past.

At that time, I was also a keen golfer and spent many hours with my friends on the golf course.

In addition, my passion for music is something that has kept me occupied and continues to bring immense joy in my life.

As the governing body member of SPIC MACAY – a society for the promotion of Indian Classical Arts, I have been actively supporting Classical Indian Music through the sponsorship of music concerts across the country.

Having been brought up in a family where music was appreciated and promoted, I was inspired to take up the sitar. World-famous musicians like Baba Alauddin Khan, Pt. Ravi Shankar and Ustad Ali Akbar Khan would stay for months in our home in New Delhi, where music soirees would be held. My mother, Sheila Bharat Ram, who also learnt to play the sitar from Pt. Ravi Shankar, was a great inspiration for me. I started learning sitar at the age of 10 and later became a disciple of Pt. Ravi Shankar. I learnt from him on-and-off over fifty years, whenever he got the time and opportunity to teach me. Part of the reason I couldn't learn continuously was that I had got deeply engrossed in the running of my company and wasn't able to spend time with him. Also, he had taken to performing all over the world and our schedules often didn't match. During the eight years that I lived in Madras, I didn't get the opportunity to learn from him at all.

Towards the beginning of the decade of 2000, I got completely disconnected from my music and didn't practice or even touch my sitar. It was just before Manju passed away that she convinced me to start playing again and to never give up my passion for the sitar. Alas, my guru, Pt. Ravi Shankar ji, also passed away at the same time.

While I have given up playing golf now, I have taken to my sitar more seriously than ever in my life before. Music, I believe is one of the greatest gifts that mankind has ever received. I play the sitar for two hours every day. My '*Riyaaz*' is therapeutic and music is my stressbuster. I gain richly from it. It also contributes deeply to a more peaceful, stable mind. To me, my music is what meditation means to most people.

Since my retirement, I have also been more deeply involved in the company's philanthropic initiatives. SRF invests heavily in its commitment to sustainable and inclusive growth in India. Today,

SRF Foundation's flagship 'Rural Education Program' covers 269 schools with 78,714+ students across 21 locations in nine Indian states. Apart from providing quality education to all, SRF Foundation also works in the areas of creating awareness of issues related to health and hygiene, natural resource management and affirmative action on a sustainable basis.

I had taken over from Manju a role as the Board Member of the Charities Aid Foundation (CAF), which is a non-government organization (NGO) that helps provide avenues for donors from companies and individuals to serve the underprivileged. I was the Chairman of CAF for 6 years, until I retired a couple of years ago.

I have also been actively involved with The Blind Relief Association, Delhi as a Trustee and took over as the Chairman of the Association, two years ago. It is an NGO working to empower visually impaired persons by imparting education and skill development training. For seventy-five years now, we have believed and will continue to believe that children and adults with visual impairment and other disabilities are invaluable human assets. They deserve the right kind of recognition and opportunity in an inclusive environment. Provision of such need-based services for the visually impaired to enable them to develop their latent talents and realize their fullest potential is what The Blind Relief Association, Delhi continuously strives for.

I am also honoured to serve CAPED – Cancer Awareness, Prevention and Early Detection Trust as its Chairperson. CAPED as the name suggests, is a platform established to create awareness about women-related cancers with a focus on cervical cancer. Besides creating awareness, CAPED also facilitates and conducts screening tests at the slums in Gurugram and across other rural parts of Haryana. At CAPED, we believe that there's a lot to be done and a lot of hearts to be healed.

I am privileged to serve two great educational institutions, the Lady Shri Ram College for Women in New Delhi and The Shri Ram Schools in Delhi NCR, as Chairman. My interactions with the young students of these institutions is what I cherish the most about my role at this stage of my life. I believe that children should be given the space to do everything and anything that they want to do. But, at the same time, through my conversations with them, I encourage the younger generation to learn about our culture, get sensitized to something that has existed in our country for thousands of years, so that they grow up to become the kind of adults who will appreciate and understand our culture.

After Manju's passing away, I reconnected with close friends. Friendships that we had established in Chennai while we were living there. We are now a small group of friends who enjoy traveling together all over the world. We try to select places we have never been to before. We go on trips anywhere from two-three weeks. Some of our most memorable ones have been trips to Latin America, where we visited Machu Picchu in Peru, the Western part of Argentina, and Brazil. The other interesting places we have visited include New Zealand, Iran and the five Stans in Central Asia. Interspersed with these foreign locations are our holidays to some lesser known hill stations in India.

Life has been good. I have watched three amazing kids grow into delightful adults, and my adorable grandchildren: most of them are teenagers now and are preparing for a number of grand life experiences. I've made music I'm proud of, I have real, true friends, who have helped me do some good things that I care deeply about. I couldn't have asked for more.

38
THE POWER OF THE AGELESS MIND
Narrated by PADMA VENKATARAMAN *to* MAYA NANDHINI

When we look at age as a mere number, rather than a milestone that reads 60, 70 or 80, the idea of staying productive and positive becomes something to look forward to, as opposed to it being a chore.

When I began contemplating doing service, I was still at a young age, and my father was a labour leader at the time. While I watched him interact with labourers, listen to their problems and come up with ways to solve their issues, it occurred to me that when I grew up, I would help people too. I thought I wanted to be a doctor then, but that did not happen. However, the seeds of service were sown at a very young age.

In 1962, at the age of 20, I moved to Vellore where my husband was the District Collector at the time. As the Collector's wife, I was involved in helping out quite a number of social welfare organizations. There was one in particular that was helping leprosy-affected people. At the time, around 58 years ago, we did not have multi-drug therapy or a cure for leprosy. A representative from the organization approached me asking for help. I did not know much about leprosy back then, but he said that he would not advise mingling with patients, but suggested that I could promote products made by them. By promoting handmade goods, I sent across a message that leprosy cannot be contracted by touching articles made by people afflicted by the disease. That was my first attempt at helping leprosy-affected people, by using my position to spread awareness.

After Vellore, I moved to Delhi for a while where I was a member of the IAS Officers' Wives Association through which I helped associations for the blind. Later, along with the All India Women's Conference, I visited old age homes in Vrindavan, for which we later helped collect funds while in Vienna. I moved in my 30s to Vienna, Austria in 1974 where I spent the next 20 years. I was, at the time, a permanent representative of the All India Women's Conference at the United Nations and was on the International NGO committee for narcotics, physically challenged, women, and the elderly. I was President of the United Nations Women's Guild, a founder-member of the Vienna Indian Women's Association (VIWA) and member and vice-president of the Austrian-Indian Association.

Once, while in India on a vacation from Vienna, I saw a few leprosy-affected people begging for alms at a traffic light. I have always felt that giving them money would only provide a short- term reprieve and will not help them in the long run. I contemplated helping them in a more permanent way, instead of handing over cash. Asking a leprosy-affected person to quit seeking alms and get a job is unfair as the stigma attached to their condition prevents them from being able to seek jobs or training. This, however, bothered me for a long time. I thought of the ways I could be helping them. I collected information at the international level and presented a paper at one of the meetings in the United Nations. Based on that, I got a project sponsored by the United Nations Food and Agriculture Organization, which was eventually implemented by the All India Women's Conference in Shahdara, situated on the border of Uttar Pradesh and New Delhi.

In 1992, as I headed into my 50th decade, I took up the Shahdara project as Honorary Project Director. In the beginning, I wasn't very sure as this was a 4,000-strong colony and had unbelievable drawbacks. At that time, I had met Anna Hazare in Delhi, who had heard about our plans. He took a look at the place and said it was going to be a big challenge and that I would need both funds and manpower to sustain development.

However, a major take away from the Shahdara project was that success breeds success. Thirty to thirty-five years ago, people affected by leprosy never dared to hope that they could be productive members of society too. Back then, the biggest challenge was convincing them that they could be. It took a long while to make them see the potential they held and that they could also be productive within their power and means.

At first I went to a small colony in Delhi and put forward my ideas to its inhabitants. Despite initial resistance, they warmed to the idea of selling products like detergent and soap, which had a higher chance of getting sold than, say, eatables. That was the first time leprosy-affected people who, until then, had to resort to begging for alms and food began earning something on their own, something by and for themselves. As the story of their success spread, more and more people came forward, asking me to help with their colonies too. When something set in motion by you begins to yield fruit and impacts others positively, it not only makes them happy, but also cheers you up. Once the challenge of convincing the members of the colony had been overcome, people approached me of their own volition. This was the case with the Shahdara colony too.

There were 20 acres of cultivable land available, which had fallen into disuse. I convinced the Food and Agricultural Organization about the merits of the land and the ways in which it could be utilized, and how members of the colony could be engaged to produce their own food. Luckily, they felt that it was a good project, too. So, in Delhi, with the help of a number of agricultural experts and institutions, the members of the colony were able to produce wheat, rice and vegetables. There was a bumper crop that year.

Alongside this, I also worked with the HOPE Foundation, an affiliate of HOPE Worldwide, to construct houses designed by Lawrie Baker for 800 families. The Delhi municipal corporation established a school and the India Tobacco Corporation set up a crèche for children under five years. I was motivated when the inhabitants of the colony, once shown the way, made the effort to make decisions on their own and thrive. The once-empty land turned into a 'Village of Hope', thriving with life and happiness, an effort brought on by hard work and a drive to accomplish positive things. There were, of course, hiccups and challenges to contend with, but they were not insurmountable. In 2001, nearly a decade after I began work on the Shahdara colony, the FAO recognized my efforts with an award for agriculture and pisciculture work toward the leprosy-affected people of the colony.

As the decades went past, the passion to do more steadily progressed. In 1997, I moved to Chennai and helmed a project geared toward the socioeconomic rehabilitation of leprosy colonies in Tamil Nadu. As the honorary director of the state-wide project in association with DANIDA (Danish International Development Agency) and WIA (Women's Indian Association), I introduced the concept of microcredit for the leprosy-affected, especially those who saw begging as their only viable option. It was an unheard of concept at the time. I had to take the people into confidence and create a rapport to make them understand that the scheme was for their benefit. The project's Revolving Fund concept ensured sustainability. In addition to it, there was a five-member committee that helped the leprosy-afflicted with self-management, empowering them to have confidence in themselves, thus restoring sustainability and self-governance.

As I reached my 60s, the last thing on my mind was the idea of slowing down. There is this notion that productivity is meant to decline the older one grows. However, I can only say that my passion to keep doing more only increased. When a person is active and keeps both their mind and body engaged, it helps them look forward to their day. And when this productivity helps and impacts others, it offers the incentive and the energy to keep moving and to keep doing better.

In 2005, along with Austrian artist Werner Dornik, I set up the Bindu School of Art in Bharatapuram Colony in Chennai for people who were afflicted by leprosy. I had met Mr. Dornik in 1993 during my stay in Vienna. He had come to India to help the leprosy-affected and expressed interest in setting up an art school in the colony. In 2007, four students of the art school held an exhibition of their work at the Kunsthalle Wein Art Gallery in Vienna. The school was a great way to introduce art as therapy to leprosy-affected people and to restore their self- confidence and self-respect through art.

All of this wasn't without its fair share of challenges, but there is always a positive side to everything and it is up to us to seek it out. It is also important to have a practical mindset to balance the positivity. Keeping in mind that all problems cannot be solved immediately is vital. Sometimes, we lose our sense of equanimity while dealing with obstacles as our focus might tend to sidle with negativity. One has to learn to spend some time for oneself, particularly in these circumstances, and from time to time, learn to unwind and take a few minutes to reflect and then get back to work recharged.

I am currently involved with several organizations – the Women's Indian Association, Srinivasa Gandhi Nilayam, Global Cancer Concern, Gandhi Peace Foundation and two boarding schools for children from leprosy-affected colonies, most of whom are first generation students. We hope to make the schools a diving point from which the children can launch their lives by going into higher education or work with self-respect and dignity.

A typical day is usually packed with meetings and decision making. In the past several months, the way we work has undergone a lot of changes in light of the pandemic that has swept through the world. Since we cannot meet people in person or conduct meetings or host events in public, it has all come down to using technology. In the initial months of the pandemic, everything practically came to a standstill, but, we familiarized ourselves with the technology necessary to keep everything on track. There are disruptions, of course, in the form of power cuts or slow internet connections, but we have learned to adapt. It is all a big challenge, but slowly things are falling into place.

Speaking of challenges, sometimes a fresh perspective is necessary to overcome them. An interesting incident that took place when I was the President of the United Nations Women's Guild comes to mind. We had collected funds for a village in Africa that was suffering from a water shortage. One of our members had gone to the village to help install a water tank to get water supply to the village so that the women there did not have to walk long distances to fetch water. Our practice was to monitor the situation and visit the locality after a couple of years to see the result and impact. When the same member visited the place after a couple of years, she was surprised to receive a lukewarm response. I believe the village had a custom of marrying off young girls and women to older men. So, the womenfolk viewed walking for water as the only way to step out and have fun. The new water tank brought water to their doorstep, curbing their activities. It was a very interesting thing that we learned that day, that what we consider to be development might not encompass the whole picture. We have to understand what people really want and what they are capable of. This is very important for chalking out any program, any plan.

As for maintaining positivity, self-reflection is important to keeping at it in a consistent manner. Every day we run, faster and faster from one problem to the next, trying to solve everything. This is probably why burnouts happen. There are only limited resources on this earth and when we use nature beyond its capacity and push ourselves far beyond our limits, we lose our balance. If a person goes after achievements with a single-minded focus, they will forget other aspects of life like the necessity of human touch or the simple pleasures of spending some time with the elderly at home or with friends. When you greet people with a simple hello or a good morning, it makes them happy even though the gesture does not require much effort. It is good practice to keep our eyes and ears open for people and for nature.

Pausing every now and then, to take a deep breath, to reflect and meditate is necessary to keep one's equanimity. Somewhere along the line, we have to stop and reflect and think about the meaning of life and what we want from it, and what we can give it in return. We should reflect on our purpose and why we do certain things and also on our contribution and why we are here on this planet. Keeping a balance is necessary to maintain a vibrant and productive life, regardless of age. We human beings have been exploiting nature without any regard for it, but now we have no other option but to slow down. An example of this is that I do not have to use a lot of paper now since I rely on technology to input and store notes, ideas and documents. There has been a distinct reduction in the usage of paper as earlier most surfaces in my workspace used to be strewn with it. I can only wonder how many trees we have saved in the past six months. A lesson to learn here is that it is possible to adapt and be more resourceful.

Through the progression of these decades, I have learned that keeping your mind and body active helps not only physically, but also mentally and emotionally. I would suggest mingling with the younger crowd. We learn so much by spending time in their company; our minds become younger when we talk to the youth. The older generation should make acquaintances and friendships outside their age group; it always has to be a mixture. Youngsters learn from the experience the older generation has to offer, and in turn, the elders can acquire new experiences and keep their minds sharp. The younger generation is open to so many new things, something which I was not while growing up.

The Global Cancer Concern, of which I am a trustee, has a cancer awareness programme that aims at encouraging children to spread cancer awareness and educate their families about it. We visit schools and talk to children about cancer, who in turn, become ambassadors. Parents listen because it is their children, and not an adult giving them advice. The programme was a success and we began collecting funds. Another project I am working on is part of the Gandhi Peace Foundation, where we are trying to inculcate Gandhian principles in schoolchildren in the form of stories. We conduct events where we have storytelling sessions for children and have printed books with stories that teach Gandhian principles. This way, children would slowly get introduced to Gandhian principles and learn positive things at a young age.

Inspiration often goes hand-in-hand with having a positive and graceful experience as you age. The Women's Indian Association celebrated its hundredth year in 2017. I collected the history of the organisation from the time of our first president Dr. Annie Besant and learned about the legislations passed by this wonderful organization for advancement of women and children – the Sarda Act which raised the marriageable age for girls, the abolition of the devadasi system which restored dignity to the art, and the ways in which women were brought to the forefront, how they participated in the national freedom movement and worked against social evils. It was an eye-opener for me, having gone through so many rich, personal histories steeped in sacrifice.

An example is Dr. Muthulakshmi Reddy. The first Indian president of the Women's Indian Association, Dr. Muthulakshmi got a scholarship and went on to attend medical college where she was the only woman student. Despite the odds, she stood first, a gold medallist. Another example of someone who embodied positivity and courage is Krishnammal Jagannathan, a freedom fighter who worked alongside Gandhiji and Vinobhaji for the Bhoodan Movement. She was frequently ill-treated by people that she came across, but worked hard on getting land for the landless.

The resilience displayed by these women is quite admirable. The more you read about them, the more inspired you get to do more, to do better. I am also in the process of reviving a magazine called *Stri Dharma*, which was started in 1917 by the Women's Indian Association. It was published till 1938 and was probably stopped during the Second World War. The magazines hold so much history, about women who fought in different ways, and what they went through to make their voices heard.

As I continue into the next decade of my life, I hope to keep finding inspiration and to also inspire those around me. I believe that keeping an open mindset, keeping oneself productive, having goals and focusing on achieving them go a long way to helping one stay young, productive and happy, regardless of one's age. As important as it is to keep moving, it is equally vital to establish balance in life and to find a sense of equanimity in ourselves, to de-stress even while focusing on responsibilities.

Every day, amid my schedule, I take some time off to unwind. I play the veena, practise meditation and pranayama. When stress takes over rational thought, it is easy to fall back into thinking that there is no light at the end of the tunnel. So, it is essential to take a step back, unwind and look at it with fresh perspective.

Reflection, retrospection and recharging are the perfect accompaniments to leading a productive existence. If we don't pause to think about our actions, their consequences and how we can improve ourselves and impact others in positive ways, we are in danger of being swallowed up by the relentless pace of life. Life exists to not only hold our achievements aloft, but also to bear the fruits of our enjoyment, and therein lies the secret to approaching new experiences with grace and positivity.

39

You Are Only Old as You Feel

Dr. Shayama Chona

I am in the twilight of life, still enjoying the sweet birds singing. It is said that sunset is followed by the dark night; Running 79 I do not see the sun of my life setting into the dark night.

People expect me to look decrepit as I age and it might even remind them that I might be soon gone, but these thoughts have never entered my mind. When I look at the mirror everyday I feel I am only growing younger.

I fear neither the wind nor the tide, I believe you are only as old as you feel. If we can remain youthful in mind and spirit, then we are young, no matter if our bodies may be growing older. As Coleridge says, "youth and I are housemates still".

Ageing encompasses every aspect of our being; body, mind and soul or physical, intellectual, spiritual and emotional, which are all based on our personal lives, experiences, thoughts and attitude.

Believe it or not, you look what you think, and it is our thoughts which keep us youthful and full of vitality, zeal, and vigour.

I believe in living life to the fullest and making each day count. My routine keeps me going, I do not even spare a single moment without productive activity. I pour my heart, mind and soul into enabling the differently abled at Tamana, and nurturing the future generations of the world studying in premier schools across the globe. My mind is always active, juggling between millions of thoughts and ideas which I endeavour to put into action. Throughout the day I am penning down tasks and ideas which I want to implement, and then working towards making them happen.

All this is possible because I take care of my mental, spiritual, and physical health. I eat little, do my yoga, daily walks, pray and spend quality time with my loved ones who are my stress busters.

Balancing mental, physical, and spiritual well being is the key to a productive life.

I follow the Gandhian philosophy, I respect all living beings including animals and birds. I am pained when I see animals and birds being slaughtered to be relished, and as a practice I am a vegetarian.

Though as a person I am not judgemental. I do not dislike anyone. I admire everyone, young or old. I believe every person is unique and has their own positives and negatives. I focus on their positives and take their mistakes as learnings. For instance, when I find someone to be rude, angry or talking ill, cursing or criticising I determine that I will refrain from such actions as I know how much hurt these can cause. I believe in non-violence. Violence can be physical or mental, as one can also be hurt by words as well. Violence is sinful and so is revenge. Forgiveness is a principle to follow as Gandhi said: "An eye for an eye would make the whole world blind."

To be happy, one has to learn to sieve out the negativities and continue to evolve as a better person: whatever qualities we admire in others we should imbibe, and what we do not like we can ensure that those traits do not become a part of our own personality.

Also, when it comes to ageing, it is our own experiences over the years with our parents, grand parents, uncles and aunts from the earlier generation which have moulded our perception that old age is synonymous with continuous doctor visits, ailments and other realities of old age. But it is in our hands as to how we perceive the impending and how we decide to lead our lives. Of course, ailments and health issues may not be that much in our control, but other aspects are.

All these thoughts that I have inherited ceaselessly, are from my parents and my upbringing. At 97 my father used to laugh heartily with sparkling eyes when he would mention how a shopkeeper tried to fool him or narrate tales of his grand children's mischief and mistakes. I learnt from him not as down-pouring of lectures or platitudes but as practical expressions of the supreme wisdom which brought good health, success, enduring happiness, love in all circumstances of life.

Another life changing experience which transformed me was the birth of my daughter, Tamana, as a cerebral palsied and a spastic baby. Eventually shock turned into faith in God and in my own ability to enable Tamana to lead a happy and productive life. Despite her delayed milestones where she began to talk and walk after the age of 9, today Tamana is a confident woman of 50, teaching as a preschool teacher at Delhi Public School Vasant Vihar since the last 20 years. I believe miracles do not just happen, we make them happen. Our only limitation is again our own thinking and attitude. Her birth taught me life is a challenge: fight it with a determination to win and success will be yours. Be brave in the face of any challenge and never give up.

If Tamana can look 20 at the age of 50, ready to take on the world, then maybe I am equally young at 78, only 2 years away from 80.

Coming back to it, it is our thinking which makes us young or old, continuously evolving our thoughts and attitudes in a positive direction keeps us mentally strong and eternally happy. Along with that I believe it is this zest for contributing towards the betterment of our children, holding on to hope, enthusiasm, optimism and forward motion which keeps one ever so youthful and raring to go with limitless energy and vitality.

While I know that I will not live forever, I seldom think of the future years.

My only prayer to God is let me go when my boots are on. I ensure that I do not lose the glory or form or lustre in my eye.

I would be foolish to ask God to give me immortality, but I am confident that my work will be immortal, and I plan to keep working as long as I can go on making the world a better place through my thoughts, words and action.

40
AGEING GRACEFULLY
LT. GENERAL (RETD.) SHANKAR PRASAD

"You don't stop laughing when you grow old,
you grow old when you stop laughing!"

– George Bernard Shaw

What is old age? With the rise in life expectancy to 76 years from the earlier 62 years, when does old age start? The term of 'old' has a totally different connotation in life today to what it did about 20 years ago! Perhaps ageing gracefully doesn't necessarily have to refer to age or appearance but rather the attitude people develop as they are growing old.

"Old man"is a term used in the Army for a Unit Commander by his officers, even though he may be 38 to 40 years of age. Some children also refer to their father as "old man" even though he may be only around 30 years of age. My "old man" retired from the Civil Services of the Government of India at a young age of 58 years and soon found a gainful position as Director in the corporate world. After his second retirement, he decided to enjoy life following the dictum, "*the key to successful ageing includes accepting changes and finding meaningful activities*". He aged gracefully and passed away at the age of 99 years without ever getting old. His "awesome family", of children, grandchildren, and great grandchildren, who also interacted with him intimately, have a lot to learn from his life.

Regular physical exercise, ideally of the nature such as walking in company, playing golf or tennis with people younger brings about a massive change in attitude towards growing old. Mental exercise must continue to remain part of physical exercise such as ideally being able to play card games or reading interesting books. My old man preferred reading books relating to his contemprory period of the Raj as well as other young and new authors to stay and feel connected with the emerging and evolving world. Participation in discussions on politics and other social issues and such activities resulted in staying connected with the newer trends in the world and within the country.

Self-esteem is a major constitutional contributor to moulding attitude. It involves creating a routine of dressing, following strict time schedules of eating meals and undoubtedly wholesome meals, not necessarily non-vegetarian but even vegetarian food which can be wholesome. Associated with this it is the consumption of alcohol which should be in moderation. It will not be out of place to say looking good and smelling good adds to self esteem and is a positive ingredient to attitude.

The above is all very good and possible for someone who has a steady income post retirement in the form of a pension or has abundant savings. However, let's look at what it's like for someone who does not have the means to do all the above activities which I have listed. Money is a great levelling factor and it can definitely help us in ageing gracefully; but for the lower income group as you age, interdependence poses a major set back. There is a kind of despondency that sets in when even his daily meals are at the behest of others within the family; his own children at times! It becomes very difficult for the individual to manage to stay upbeat and to manage life on his own. He turns into a child once again, looking inwards to his children to accept him till his dying days. There is no self-esteem left there, neither is there any independence left, all money seems to have dried up and he is at the mercy of the children. Obviously he is not going to be ageing very gracefully. He is now just waiting to be consumed by death which is a sorry state of affairs, but something which he just has to accept, as nothing can be done about this. Old age homes are now becoming the norm these days. Children feel they've done their duty, but does it help the elderly to age gracefully?

All this goes on if he is physically fit but woe betide if he falls sick; paralytic/ surgically incapacitated or gets a life threatening disease like cancer. With no money at his disposal, and no landed property for raising money, he just lives on the sympathy of the family. My mother's prayers to the Lord were always to keep her limbs functioning and not become a liabilty on anyone! Family disputes and petty jealousies amongst siblings and clash of interest within one's own children can be very demoralising.

However, notwithstanding the above, taking an active part in the affairs of the family in an advisory capacity, helping take care of the youngsters, supervising homework of the school going kids, helping with the household chores, helping in the community work, can help in being accepted and keeping up the self esteem, thus keeping alive the will to live. Religion can also play a major role whereby all energies are expended in praying, keeping mental tension at bay and also helping to pass time which hangs on the individual.

One needs to always remember to "Count your blessings not your wrinkles".

41
OLD AGE
KAMLA BHASIN

बुज़ुर्गयित
मेरे बालों की सफ़ेदी
दखिाती है मेरा अन्दरूनी नखिार
मेरे चेहरे की झुर्रयिाँ
दर्शाती हैं मेरे तजुर्बात के उभार।
बार बार मेरा भूलना बताता है
कमिेरी hard disc है अब भर गई।
चलने की रफ़्तार में आई कमी
कहती है, अब जल्दी नहीं कहीं भी जाने की।
सो, खुश हूँ मैं
बुढ़ापे की इन नशिानयिों के साथ।
जवानी की बेचैनयिाँ
अपनी जगह ठीक थीं
मगर, बूज़ुर्गीअ तका ये ठहराव,
ये गहराई भी कोई कम नहीं।

– कमला भसीन

The silver of my hair
Reflects my inner glow.
The ridges on my face
My experiences show.
My forgetfulness says
My hard disk is full.
The slowing of my pace
Knows no binding pulls.
So, happy am I
With these signs of age.
The passions of youth
Were good in their time,
But the calm depth of age
Is just as beautiful.

(Translation by Meenakshi Paul)

Through this poem I am sharing what I feel about signs of old age in my body. The law of nature says that if anyone lives long, s/he must age. Hence ageing or getting old is inevitable, but how we age is up to each one of us.

I am 74 and I am ageing, but I have no idea how a 74-year old person should feel. After all, I have never been 74 before. I feel the same as I did when I was 50 or 60. Yes, my body is different; hair is greyer, face has more wrinkles, body is not as agile, but it still does whatever I want to do – i.e., walks, does yoga, lifts things, jumps and dances around, bends, uses ladders, cycles, drives, and so on..

This Is Who I Am

Maybe it will help you to understand me better if I share with you some basic facts about my life. I live in Delhi with my 40 year old son, Jeet, who has been very severely challenged since he was about a year old. He is quadriplegic, meaning all four limbs of his do not work; he has no motor function, head control and speech.

This means he cannot do anything for himself. He needs full time care. He is big and quite heavy, so I have not been able to pick him up, bathe him, etc., for many years. Because he cannot speak and has no motor function, he cannot tell us what he needs, or what is hurting or bothering him. To care for him and also me, I have four full time people. Two of them are a couple and they have a five-year old son, Suansh. All seven of us live in a flat, like a family. They look after me and I try my best to look after them. It is because of their love and care that my son is alive and well, and I have the freedom and possibility to continue to do my work.

I had a daughter, Meeto. She was doing a PhD in Oxford when she committed suicide. She was suffering from clinical depression. She was only 27 years old.

After 35 years of marriage, my partner and I divorced, because he got involved with a woman who was 35 years younger than him and had a child with her, without marrying her.

It has not been easy to deal with all these adversities but, to the extent that I have managed. I think I have managed because of the support of my siblings and friends, and because I was economically independent and had meaningful, satisfying work. In addition, wise people like the Buddha and couplets like the one below by Maulana Hafiz have guided me. An Iranian friend of mine had this couplet written in beautiful calligraphy for me, to show me the way to take and go.

Zeereshamsheereghamaash
Raqskonaanbauyaadraft

– Maulana Hafiz

This couplet says: *Now that you have no choice but to go under the sword of separation, you might as well go dancing.*

This is what I have been trying to do. Also, I know that this is what my daughter Meeto would expect of me, nothing less. My dancing around also pleases my son Jeet and I also prefer it to spending a sad miserable life. I think, Jeet also keeps me young at heart. He is a permanent child and I have to play the fool all the time to make him laugh, to sing for and with him, do funny things which make him happy. Didn't the Buddha tell that heartbroken mother whose child passed on, that there is no home in the world without death and adversity? So, why not me?

Are We Just Our Perishable Bodies?

Now back to ageing… For me the question is, am I just my body? Do just the changes in my body decide whether I am 'ageing' or not,and how I should feel and behave?

I do not know the answers to these questions. I don't know how one feels old. I am also not particularly wiser than before, although I have seen a lot of life. I still make mistakes. There are so many things I still do not know. I remain a student, a Taalib, a Sikh or Shishya. I am happy to learn from anyone, older people, younger people, village people, city people, so-called educated and uneducated people, anyone. This desire to keep learning means, I always have something to do. My brain is always ticking. I am forever curious. I love to meet and know people. I ask questions, so many questions that sometimes people think I am nosey. I don't think I am nosey. I think because I consider people important, precious, unique, I wish to know them; I want them to know I am interested in them, I care about them.

Maybe I do not feel old because I have not 'REtired' from my work. Actually, I am not even 'tired' of my work, forget about Retiring. Even at 74 I have not retired because in the activist, civil society work I do, there is no retirement age. What an absolute blessing. We can keep doing things we enjoy, till the body feels or falls dead.

Actually, I am not even sure if I will die. Maybe I am ***not*** just my body. May be there is a soul and that is the real me and I will soar away, lightly, without the weight and shortcomings of this body. Who knows? I don't know. I will find out when the transition takes place, but then I will not be able to tell you what it is. What a pity. Sorry folks!

If Work Is Worship, Life Is Youthful

Maybe I do not feel old or as if I am ageing because I love what I do. I have always felt blessed to have work which never seems like work. My work is also my hobby and to be paid to do your hobby or passion is the best thing which can happen to anyone. I cannot even imagine how people work only to make a living, only to earn. How do they spend a whole life doing something which they do not like or value? Is that livelihood or deadlihood?

I feel, if we have exciting work to do, we do not sit around with an empty mind inviting the devil to play around in our head. This is specially so if our work is connected to some human values like human rights, equality, justice, truth and if our work is to help others. Shantideva, the Buddhist practitioner and scholar, said a long time ago that "All the suffering there is in this world arises from wishing our self to be happy. All the happiness there is in this world arises from wishing others to be happy." And, when we are happy, we feel young.

Giving is the key to successful and youthful living.

For me, there has never been a divide between work and leisure or work and re-creation. My work has never tired or destroyed me to make me seek re-creation. My work has been re-creating me. To give an example, part of my work has been to write songs and slogans and rhymes for children, which challenge gender and other inequalities. I have also been creating posters and banners. All this is exciting, creative, fun. So, for me there has not been a difference between free time and bondage time.

Friendships, Connections and Love Are Tonics for Youthfulness

Since 1975, my work has been to organize collective learning opportunities and networking in South Asia and other countries, first through the UN and then through informal civil society networks. This has involved a lot of travel. Every journey took me to friends in whose homes I stayed. Seldom did I stay in hotels. This is why I have enjoyed every bit of travel in the course of my official duties because it was always friendship travel too. I don't only ***think*** but I ***know*** that love, friendship and connections are effective tonics to keep us young, vibrant and radiant. Love is youthful, youth is love. Age does not matter. Isn't the art of loving the art of youthful, exciting living?

Strong and Healthy Body Is Beautiful and Youthful

I have been into outdoor activities and sports since my childhood. We grew up in villages of Rajasthan and it was difficult for my parents to keep me indoors. I was fortunate that my parents did not lock me in because I was a girl. I ran, climbed trees, played *gilli danda*, *kanchey* or marbles, *satolia* or *pitthu*, hockey and cricket with homemade bats and hockey sticks. On rented bicycles, I learnt cycling and, when I was 17 or 18 years of age, learnt to drive a scooter on other people's scooters because we did not own a scooter. In my childhood I could beat most boys in most games, and in the 50s and 60s boys had not been taught by patriarchal media that playing with girls was not cool.

In the Government college and university I went to in Jaipur, I was the General Captain, meaning the head of all sports. For me beauty was the strength and suppleness of the body and not the market defined, beauty which could be achieved only with purchased cosmetics. I have always tried to have a healthy and fit body, and for that I did sports and later yoga. Even today I do yoga regularly and keep fit. I think this has kept me active and youthful.

Going with the Flow

I think I have been flowing with the flow of life, going where life has been taking me, accepting what I could not change; not fretting too much. Yes, during difficult times I felt sad and cried heartily and openly when it was too much, but moved on. I have tried to accept both sadness and joy, darkness and light, day and night because they always come in pairs and one cannot choose just one of them.

Truly, age for me has been just a number. Unlike many women or people, I have not given undue importance to looking a certain way and living according to all the gender norms. So, I have never removed my body hair to look *kamsin* or young in years; I have never colored my cheeks or lips to look youthful, never dyed my hair which started greying very early. I have never hesitated to tell my age or to pretend I was younger. I have always felt and said that this pressure on girls and women to always look pretty and young and that too defined by the cosmetic and other industries, is most oppressive and harmful.

I feel every age and every phase of life is unique and we need to accept and enjoy all of them. I wrote these couplets to express what I feel:

Zindagi kaa har daur anootha hai
Maine har daur ka maza loota hai.
Umda zindagi wo naheen jo lambee waali hai
Maine to har lamhain me Zindagi daali hai.

(Every phase of life is unique.
I have enjoyed the uniqueness of every phase.
Good life is not that which is long,
I have lived every moment fully and poured life in to it)

The Child in Me Is Alive and Kicking

I think we do not feel old if the child in us is alive. My body has seen many summers but the child in me is still there. Five years ago, I spent two full days flying kites with a man friend who is as old as me. During this year's monsoon season, I played around in the rain with my grandson. For and with my son and grandson I keep writing and reciting poems. Sometime seeing my pranks and being irritated by them, my daughter asked, "Amma, tell me who is the child in our relationship?"

In response I told her, "You tell me why **you** behave like an old woman sometimes?"

To highlight the need for everyone to be childlike, I actually wrote a long poem, which was published by Jagori as a book with beautiful illustrations with the title *Ulti Sulti Amma*. This came after I wrote *Ulti Sulti Meeto*, which was about a girl. People who nurture their inner child remain curious, loving, exciting and young in every way, even bodily young.

Humour and Laughter Keep Us Youthful

I am very serious about laughter because I know it is very healthy; it spreads good cheer and if we laugh with others rather than laugh at others, it keeps us happy and vibrant. I don't think feminists like me would have survived in this patriarchal and terribly anti-feminist society without humour. Laughter is an essential ingredient for a happy youthful life. There is no limit on its dosage. You can have as much of it as you want. Not only do I use and create every opportunity to laugh and make others laugh, but have, along with my friend Bindia Thapar, created two books on feminist humour, published by Jagori, Delhi. I have used humour in many of my songs and I am happy to report that my funny songs are very popular and they cheer everyone up. I am very glad that many yoga practitioners have been popularising laughing yoga and laughter clubs have emerged all over. Through our smiles and laughter, let us ensure that we bring happiness wherever we go and not whenever we go. I hope you are clever enough to understand my joke. Ha Ha!

Living in the Present Moment

I have benefitted greatly by the Buddha's wisdom, "The only thing which does not change is change", and his advice to always live in the present moment. When I was in my fifties, I went for a ten day Vipassana meditation course. That proved to be most helpful. That ten day long *maun* or silence, watching my breath and thoughts for 11 hours a day; that deep immersion in to myself proved to be transformative. It taught me to accept changes, both good and bad; to realize that our bodies are perishable, they are changing every moment and moving towards ultimate bodily death. Once you understand this then you accept all ages; you do not consider any age to be better than the other. I also learnt that death is the only certain thing, although we do not know when it will happen. Anything that is born will die. I think I managed to internalise some of these messages and Vipassana helped me accept the biggest and most painful loss of my 27-year old daughter.

The Mahamritunjaya Mantra has also helped me accept bodily ageing, fragility and the ultimate death. In Sanskrit it is, "*Om triyambakam, yajaamahe, sugandhim, pushtivardhanam; Urvaruk miv bandhanaan mrityor mukshiya maamritaat*". To me the main message of the mantra is that the only way to overcome death is to accept it and to be free of the fear of death. Similarly, the only way to age gracefully is to accept ageing and the fact that our bodies are ever changing and perishable. Also, we human beings need to accept that if we are living longer today, we have to accept the problems that come with old age.

The practice of mindfulness, popularized by the Buddhist Master Thich Nhat Hanh, has also helped me understand the monkey nature of our mind so as to live better. Living mindfully means, living in the present moment; being alive all the time; engaging deeply with those around us. Developing an attitude of gratitude has also been a blessing. Appreciating all that I have and recognizing all the relationships which have enriched my life, has helped me live well. Living mindfully with an attitude of gratitude has helped me appreciate and enjoy the ordinary things of life; a nice roasted *bhutta* (corn) or *shakarqandi* (sweet potato), a nice hot water *baalti* bath, an unexpected phone call from a dear one, a beautiful tree….. This attitude has helped me realize that life is too precious to be wasted on silly quarrels, misunderstandings, stupid worries. It is better to spend time appreciating people, affirming them and bonding with them.

Toxic and painful relationships, I believe, make us unhappy. They eat us up from the inside. It is best to distance ourselves from toxic relationships if there is no chance of them improving. We should try and keep the others happy and fun. This couplet has been a good guide for me:

Kuchh is tarah hamne zindagi ko aasaan kar liya
Kisi se maafi maang lee, kisiko maaf kardiya.

(I have made my life easy
by apologising to some and pardoning some.)

Humility and simplicity are other traits I have found useful for living and growing old gracefully.

I will end my reflections about ageing by quoting from a meaningful poem on this theme I found on social media. The writer is unknown to me but much appreciated, and from my feminist book titled *Laughing Matters*, published by Jagori, Delhi:

I don't complain
About getting old.
Just think of all the people
Who are denied this privilege.
Growing old can be a
Wonderful Adventure, if
We remember that the keyword is GROWING.

And I conclude with this lovely poem which expresses everything I want to say in just a few words.

Umra ka badhnaa to dastoor-e-jahaan hai
Mahsoos na karein, to badhtee kahaan hai?
Umra ko agar haraanaa hai to shauq zinda rakhiye
Ghutne chalein na chalein, mann udta parindaa rakhiye.
Mushkilon kaa aana to part of life hai
Unmein se hanskar baahar aana Art of Life hai.

Translation:

The increase in our age is a law of nature,
If we refuse to pay attention to ageing,
how can ageing increase?
If you wish to defeat age, nurture some hobbies.
Even if your knees do not work,
keep your heart flying like a bird.
Facing adversities is part of life
Smiling through them is the Art of Life.

42
REFLECTIONS FROM THE PAST
DR. MOHINDER SINGH

"It is said that the best way to spend your old age is to relive your childhood."

(Popular saying)

I was born in a hilly hamlet named Durakhshail in the Haripur frontier district of West Panjab (Pakistan) on the 23rd of November, 1941. Only child of my parents (not because of family planning but because of high infant mortality rate) Jagjit Kaur and Hari Singh, I moved to the princely city of Patiala during the partition in a train guarded by the Gurkha police which was considered neutral when the Punjab police got divided on communal lines as a result of partition. After two days of arduous journey in a packed compartment without any food or water, we reached Patiala railway station in heavy downpour in the month of August 1947 and took shelter under a shed on the platform. When the next train arrived we were pushed so hard by the new crowd that we reached the road without much effort. Not knowing where to go we kept on walking till we found a make-shift shelter for the refugees in the *Gaushala* where on arrival we were served food by the volunteers. Hurray! I spent my first night in Independent India in a barn meant for feeding cows!

Thanks to democracy and education, which empowers ordinary citizens, I entered the same city sixty-seven years later as a State Guest when I was invited by the Punjabi University to deliver a 37th convocation address with the Governor of Panjab presiding over the function. On arrival in the circuit house, I was presented a guard of honour by the state police because of my quasi-judicial position as Member of the National Commission for Minority Educational Institutions. The focus of my address was on the importance of democracy and education. Democracy demolished the Mall Road which divided the feudal aristocracy of Patiala who lived in mansions and *hoi polloi* in the *mohallas* on the other side of the Mall. Education empowers the poor to compete and occupy positions which were the privilege of children from thw aristocracy up to now.

Coming back to the story, after a few day's stay in the *Gaushala* we started looking for a house of our own. There was no problem in finding a house as many of the Muslim males were mercilessly killed by the Hindu and Sikh fanatics and their women raped and either killed or sent to refugee camps. This was being done because of provocation by so-called religious leaders as part of the 'revenge' for similar acts of madness committed by Muslim fanatics on other side of the border. One incident which has got embedded in my memory as a child is that of a naked swollen body of a woman right at the entrance of the house which we were going to occupy. Surely this woman was raped either by Hindu or a Sikh fanatic as Muslim men were either being killed or running to safe havens. This was the incident which greatly motivated me to fight against communal violence for the rest of my life.

I lost my father a year after reaching Patiala. My mother was so lost in finding ways and means to bring me up and could hardly think of sending me to school. I envied children of my age who were going to school carrying books and a slate, and I longed to join them. One day, without telling my mother. I accompanied my cousin and reached the Government Primary School near Sheranwalan Gate, Patiala. When the teacher questioned my cousin as to who was this 'intruder', I quickly replied that I wanted to join the school. The teacher asked me my name, and other details, I got stuck on the issue of age as I did not carry any birth certificate (in fact no one carried any authentic documents those days). My age was decided in a rather interesting manner. The teacher asked me to stand with my back on the wall in the centre and asked a boy who looked younger and another who looked elder. One was five and other was seven, so I was arbitrarily declared to be six years old. But how the teacher decided that I was born on 23rd of November, 1941, still remains a mystery.

It was during school days that I learnt interesting stories about Patiala *Trimurti* – three legendary figures in the town who greatly influenced me in life. And there were Dr. Ganda Singh, eminent historian, Dr. Khushdeva Singh well-known specialist in chest diseases and Shri Dasondhi Ram, popularly known as 'Birji'. There was anxiety in my mind to have *Darshan* of this *Trimurti*, but was told by my teacher it is not possible to meet them. One day we had an interesting experience when we were playing marbles in the school ground during the recess. Suddenly a man with soiled clothes, unshaved beard and wearing old slippers appeared on the scene. He asked us to stand up and started slapping us without any rhyme or reason. Before we could realise what had happened, our headmaster appeared on the scene and touched the feet of this 'stranger'. He rebuked us for wasting our time in playing marbles which, he said, was *Buri Baat*, a bad habit and advised us to look around the area for waste papers and peanut peels. He pointed towards the empty tin boxes fixed on the wall with Use Me written on them and advised us to pick-up the waste around the school campus and deposit in the tin. Later when we asked our class teacher who this person was and why our headmaster was scared of him, we were told this was the legendary figure you were longing to meet. An educated man from the well-to-do Kapoor family of the town Birji was employed as a high official by the Maharaja of Patiala. On watching the sufferings of the poor, especially those suffering from incurable diseases and were disowned by their families, he started looking after them. In the process he would often get late for his office, and sometime later he was so engrossed in his mission that he would often forget to attend his office. One day on a complaint made by his immediate superior to Maharaja Yadavendra Singh, the then ruler of Patiala State, he was called to explain his irresponsible behaviour and was warned that if he did not mend his ways he would be dismissed from the state service. The Maharaja also told him that once being thrown out from the state service, he would find it impossible to get any job. Unmoved, Birji politely told the Maharaja that he was not worried about an alternative job as he was already gainfully employed. The Maharaja was surprised at the reply and asked him the details of his 'other employment'. On learning that Birji was busy serving the destitute and disposing off unclaimed dead bodies, the Maharaja was greatly moved and asked Birji to continue with his mission and the state would send his monthly salary to his home with a rider. The Maharajah also instructed that when the ruler passed away Birji should be first among the pallbearers. For me Birji has been a source of inspiration.

After passing my primary class, I joined the newly opened Government Multipurpose School in Patiala. It was here that I met a teacher, Sardar Pritam Singh who was another great influence on me. As a Scout Master he would advice us to perform one good act a day like helping a blind or disabled person to cross the road, carrying an injured man to the hospital or other little acts of service. One day when my cousin and I were returning from Chandigarh by bus, the bus stopped suddenly at the city entrance. We got down and noticed that a man with a motorcycle had met with an accident and nobody was present to take care of him. Remembering the advice of our scout master we decided to miss the bus and looked for help. Cars on the road were rare those days, but we were fortunate to find a family travelling by car to Patiala. We managed to stop the car and requested the family to take the injured person to Rajendra Hospital in Patiala. We were careful in taking out his wallet which contained his visiting card.

We also removed his gold bangle and watch to prevent any loss when he was unconscious in the hospital. One of us managed to locate his family and inform them. Next day when we narrated this incident to our Scout Master he took us to the Headmaster to be congratulated This act of ours was narrated to all the students during the morning assembly next day.

When I joined the college I found that our Principal Dr. Ganda Singh was my Scout teacher's father. Sometimes he would advise students to practise simple values taught by Guru Nanak. He would exhort all students to shun ostentation and when the time came to go in for a simple marriage ceremony to be performed before sunrise called *Amritvela* after recitation of the *Asa Di Var.* After passing my graduation examination. I went on to do my post graduation in History and took up my first teaching job in Baring Union Christian College, Batala, run by the Presbytarian Church of North America. It was during my stay in this college that I learnt how to respect women. I watched my two colleagues in the History Department, Dr. Hew McLeod and Dr. John Webster, helping their wives in the kitchen, doing laundry and other chores which were considered by our Punjabi society as belonging to the female domain. There I learnt many good values, one of them being family get-togethers in the college campus where every teacher had to join with family. When my colleague Dr. Hew McLeod noticed that I had not taken my mother with me, he asked me the reason for her absence. My simple reply was she would not be able to socialise as she was not conversant with English which was the common medium of communication used in such gatherings with a large presence of American faculty and visiting Fulbright fellows. Dr. McLeod, who was working on the Janamsakhi tradition and was fluent in written and spoken Punjabi, accompanied me to our flat in the campus and spoke to my mother in fluent Punjabi and took her to the family club. Interestingly, the Principal of the college, Dr. C. H. Loehlin, who had done his Ph. D. on 'Sikhs and their Scripture', also spoke fluent Punjabi. At the end of the academic session, one of my colleagues, who later became my brother-in-law, asked me my plans during the vacation. I was frank with him and conveyed to him my mother's fears that I would marry one of the Fulbright scholars and get converted to Christianity. In a casual talk he asked me what I looked for in my prospective spouse. I had very few requirements just a tall lady with a post graduate degree in English Literature so that she could take up a job and make our married life financially smooth. Lo and behold he invited me to his house for tea and introduced me to my would be bride who met my requirements. And the week after we arranged a simple marriage in which I kept my promise of an ostentation-free ceremony given to my teacher Dr. Ganda Singh. At the simple engagement event, I was presented with a *Gutka* (Sikh Prayer book), small *Kirpan*, some sweets and a wedding ring and gold *Kara*. While I did not make any fuss during the ceremony soon after I removed the ring and the gold *Kara* and put them back in the case given by the jeweller. Accepting any gold items was against the advice of my teacher. To the objection of some of my relatives I told them that if our marriage was to last it will last even without a gold ring. If it was to break, it will break even with a diamond ring. Fortunately we have lived happily for more than five decades facing life's ups and downs together. Coming back to marriage ceremony, a date was fixed for a simple ceremony in the house of Principal of the State College of Patiala, a relative of my in-laws. An evening before the marriage I sent a message that I wanted to meet their family elder to discuss some urgent issues. This might have created a panic in their family thinking that the groom had a list of demands. During the meeting that evening I spelt out my demands – no tent to be fixed for the ceremony, *Anand Karaj* will be performed early morning and there would be no lunch. Instead after the *Anand Karaj* we will have tea on the same dining table which was being used by the family with three chairs to be added. For the priest who was to perform the *Anand Karaj* I made a personal request not to deliver any sermons during the ceremony, as I knew the Sikh

Rahit Maryada (Code of Conduct) better than him. As settled, we did not carry any dowry items except her school, college and university Degrees which would give us a dowry every month. And this served us well as I retired without a pension and medical facilities while my wife gets a pension every month and I am dependent on her for the medical facilities of the Delhi Government as a retired school principal.

When after the marriage we entered our home, my cousin, who was quite upset by my unconventional ways, gave us a cold reception. To make my wife comfortable in her 'new home' I entered the kitchen and I made tea for her (a practice which was followed by my colleagues in the Baring College). This really offended my cousin who angrily stated, 'You have brought us dishonour' (*Tu Sada Nak Katwa Ditta Hai*). After tea together we played a game of scrabble. Noticing that my wife was not feeling at home in her 'new home'. I decided to move to Baring College without spending the rest of our summer vacation in our Patiala home.

After serving for two years in Baring College, Batala, we moved to Delhi where I got a teaching job in the Khalsa College, University of Delhi, and my wife got a job as Senior Teacher of English (PGT) in a school. It was during our stay in Delhi that we were gifted with two beautiful daughters and life moved on. Some years later when Dr. Amrik Singh was appointed as Vice-Chancellor of Punjabi University, Patiala, I along with some young academics from Delhi, moved to Patiala as the new Vice-Chancellor wanted to induct young blood into the History Department. A few years later I was invited to take over as Director of Guru Nanak Foundation, New Delhi. It was here that I came in close contact with Mrs. Mohini Giri. A well-known name in the social circles of the national capital, Mrs. Giri was involved with many organisations of social service including the War Widows' Association which was located on the same road quite close to Guru Nanak Foundation. I discovered Mrs. Giri's spirit of service during the aftermath of anti-Sikh riots in November 1984. With a view to providing relief and moral support to the unfortunate widows of the riots, Mrs. Giri came out in open support of victims of riots at the hands of anti-social elements supported by some political elements. Late one evening she entered Guru Nanak Foundation's compound with unfortunate widows and their children and loudly almost ordered me to open the offices and the auditorium where these victims could be camped till the situation became normal. When I tried to argue that I need permission from my management she expressed her anger saying, "These are sisters and daughters of the Sikh families whose male members have been killed by the ruffians, and as head of a Sikh institution you need to provide them shelter as they were feeling insecure in the building where they were housed."

She almost commanded me to arrange recitation from the Granth Sahib so as to provide some mental relief to them. I had no courage to disobey her orders and we tried our best to provide the facilities as suggested by her. In the next few days, I also accompanied her to relief camps in areas where no cars could enter to provide relief material. What really moved me was that her young daughter, who was suffering from cold and fever, was also asked to accompany us. Thereafter we developed some bonding and I started treating her as my elder sister and would generally obey her command during various programmes at home and abroad.

Inspired by the example of Mrs. Giri, we started a project of social service, though I must admit we were not successful, for want of experience and a social network. One day while passing through Rohini with a friend, I noticed a Sikh flag in Sector 16-J of the colony. I asked him if there was a Gurdwara but but he had no answer. Since I was curious to know I visited that colony again and was told this was called 'Sardar Colony' because some of the widows of 1984 riots were given small quarters by the V. P. Singh government. While most of us knew about the settlement of war widows in Tilak Vihar, this colony was unknown and consequently remained neglected. I discussed this with

Dr. J. S. Neki, who was General Secretary of our institution and with his support, we decided to open a dispensary which was named Bibi Bhani, after the daughter of 3rd Guru Amardas who is known in Sikh history for her service. My wife who was then teaching in a school, motivated some of her colleagues and together they started teaching children in the area after their school hours. With some donations, from Dr. Neki and other friends, and medicines being provided ex gratia by Bhai Mohan Singh of Ranbaxy, both school and dispensary started functioning very well. But upon my wife's retirement from the Principalship of the school, to continue managing it became a little difficult. Fortunately, some well-meaning enthusiastic friends came to our rescue and took over our project which is running very well, though under a different name.

My association with Mrs. Giri continued even after I moved from Guru Nanak Foundation to the newly established Institute of Panjab Studies in Bhai Vir Singh Sahitya Sadan in the Gole Market institutional area. On my suggestion Dr. Manmohan Singh, Chairman of the Sadan nominated Mrs. Giri onto the governing body of our institution. It was with the active support of Dr. Amrik Singh, Mrs. Giri, Dr. Nirmala Deshpande and other well-meaning Members of the Governing Body that Sadan was able to arrange many workshops and seminars including an International seminar on the Guru Granth Sahib and the Guru's context which was inaugurated by Dr. Manmohan Singh, then Prime Minister of India in the Vigyan Bhawan on 30th October, 2005, and another international seminar on Pluralistic Vision in Guru Granth Sahib which was inaugurated by Mrs. Pratibha Devi Singh Patil, then Hon'ble President of India, in Vigyan Bhavan on December, 16, 2010.

However, I discovered the most practical form of social service during my participation in Annual Peace Prayer arranged by Rome-based Community of Sant'Egidio founded by Prof. Andrea Riccardi. As most of the young couples in Italy, in fact most of Europe do not raise their own families, they spend their weekends attending to the elder citizens in their vicinity. The wife will go to one home and the husband to another, updating senior citizens telephone numbers, paying their pending bills, and doing their laundry. This community has become a powerful movement in whole of Italy and the neighbouring countries. I do not remember how and on whose recommendation, I was invited to attend a peace conference in Milan in September1993 to represent the Sikh religion. When I was asked to speak, I noticed there were no women on the dais. While talking about Sikh tradition, I mentioned that Guru Nanak, founder of Sikh religion emphasised equality between men and women and his most powerful message contained in the Sikh holy book is, "Why deny equal respect to a woman, as it is she who gives birth to the King, highest authority in those times?" I made a reference to equality in all traditions in theory but not in practice and I made a pointed reference that the holy mother who had given birth to Christ is not being celebrated. This created some commotion which was noticeable during the lunch break, but I was happy to notice support for my suggestion among the youth. In the subsequent peace conferences called in Rome, Assisi, Florence and other places, women were invited and shared the dais with interfaith leaders from various traditions. I am glad to notice that Pope Francis, present head of the Catholic Church has introduced many overdue reforms in the Church.

During the Parliament of World's Religions called in Chicago, Cape Town, Barcelona, Salt Lake City, Melbourne and Toronto, there was increasing and active participation of women in all sessions of the Parliament.

It is a matter of satisfaction that due to dedicated leaders like Mrs. Mohini Giri, more and more women are participating in various social welfare activities. I was especially happy to notice that through the efforts of Mrs. Giri, culture of Mahadham (a shelter home for aged women disowned by their families) is fast catching up. With the emergence of nuclear families, old and aged are feeling neglected. The problem of loneliness has become acute especially during the present challenge from the

Corona pandemic. The advice to observe precautions should not be interpreted to mean a disconnect with elders in the family. Especially now, when because of old age, senior citizens cannot move out and socialise, it is all the more important for the younger members of the family to look after the elders, in keeping with the age-old tradition of India.

Here I would like to share an interesting experience. The Tibet House in Delhi has organized for some years a tree plantation to mark the birthday of His Holiness, the Dalai Lama. I suggested to the organisers that instead of planting trees in the Lodhi Road institutional area we ought to plant trees in a park in Rohini where there were no trees. They welcomed my suggestions and accordingly I advised the society being run by my wife to make needed arrangements. We located a park near the colony, arranged for volunteers to make the pits, got different types of trees from the nursery and arranged water supply. We were not aware that governmental permissions had to be sought for improving our environment. Some horticulture inspectors appeared on the scene and threatened that we would be arrested for trespassing. We tried to get permission through the local Member of the Legislative Assembly, but were told that it was not clear as to whether the park belonged to Slum Wing of DDA or the North Delhi Municipal Corporation. Therefore, we were advised to drop the idea of tree planting. Not knowing how to cross this last-minute hurdle created by the inspector 'Raj', we approached Mrs. Kiran Bedi, who was then serving as Inspector General (Prisons) in Delhi and was an admirer of the Dalai Lama. She appreciated our plan of tree plantation and happily agreed to be the Chief Guest at the impromptu function b. To everyone's surprise the police inspector of the area who had threatened us with arrest, saluted us when we entered the park accompanied by Mrs. Kiran Bedi. During the brief impromptu function Mrs. Bedi not only planted the trees but also addressed the young boys and girls in the area and in the presence of the police and other officials connected with the maintenance of the park asked them to answer a question, "*Park kis ka hai?*" (To whom does the park belong?) and the children would answer, "*Park bachon ka hai*" (It belongs to children). She instructed the officials to ensure that the trees planted by her in the presence of young boys and girls were watered regularly. It was because of Mrs Giri's inspiration that my wife and I are able to so social work.

43
Age Is Just a Number
Zena Sorabjee

Many times I have heard from people that "age is just a number." I often thought about the phrase as I grew older. I began to realize how true it was. As the years passed by, I did not feel older than the previous year. It began to dawn on me that one is as old as one feels. I did not feel that age was creeping up on me except for the few occasions when some people asked me my age and I had to tell them that I would not look upon being 85 again.

By the grace of God, I have led a physically and mentally fit life. Maybe there is longevity in the family, having three brothers, all over 90. But I think it is also due to the attitude one has towards life and death. My mother always taught us that one's life was meant to be of use to society, so we tried our best to lead a life in consonance with that principle. We also were convinced that death was not something to grieve about, it was just a transition from one life to another better life:

> I have made death a messenger of joy to thee,
> wherefore dost thou grieve?
>
> – Baha'u'llah.

From childhood, I had no interest in cards or mahjong, so I did not resort to those in my old age, which I find occupies many of the older women around me. As a young girl, when I was about 12 years old, my mother, encouraged my sister and myself to teach literacy to young adults who were tribals living in a colony near to us. So we put up a black board on the terrace and had quite a few participants in our class. This was the beginning of my interest in education which I was inspired to take up seriously in my old age. As a Baha'i by religion, I understand that education is of primary importance, and to educate even one person, brings blessings. Also, the principle of gender equality is considered a spiritual principle in the Baha'i Faith, and therefore the education of girls needs to be promoted: women, having formerly been deprived, must now be allowed equal opportunities with men for education and training.

There must be no difference in their education. Until the reality of equality between man and woman is fully established and attained, the highest social development of mankind is not possible, as it says in Baha'i Writings.

Seeing as millions of girls grew up without education, I got involved in the setting up of an Institution called Barli in Indore. This was inhouse training for illiterate adult women between the ages of 18 and 30. The Institute provided accommodation and food for six months' training, during which they learnt to read and write, and develop an income-generating skill. At first the parents refused to send the girls, but with gentle persuasion and showing that the girls would be in a safe environment, they cautiously sent their daughters. Our education system was based on functional literacy. They learnt words from day one, which they could easily associate with, for instance *naam* (name), the discussion of which also removed prejudice of names of people belonging to different religions. The attitude towards girls of different castes slowly began to change, and they were guided to believe that all are creatures of the same God.

This, therefore, was to be my direction as age crept upon me. I took to the field of education. The subject which interested me the most was history. This interest was, strangely, developed in me by my semi-literate grandmother. She would be confined in bed, and request me as a young girl, to read to her. She would choose the book, and it would invariably be a book on early Baha'i history. As I read page after page of the history of the early followers of Baha'u'llah, the Founder Prophet of the Baha'i Faith, and the sufferings that Baha'u'llah underwent, to teach the people of the oneness of mankind, the oneness of religion, and the oneness of God, I was hooked on history. Many years later, I wrote a book on the subject.

In my middle age, I was mostly occupied in travelling all over India and Asia to visit Baha'i communities and help them in the many educational institutions which Baha'I had set up in rural areas. The emphasis in these schools was always on character building so that the children would grow up to become adults who would be able to make moral choices. The need for this was deeply felt as many parts of the world suffered from exploitation and corruption.

We needed a new race of men and women who would be upright citizens of a country. It was inspiring to see large numbers of girls coming to the schools as the parents had accepted that gender equality was a spiritual principle and was to be the norm.

As my travels grew less and I retired from active life, I plunged myself into what has become a passion with me. At the age of 75, I felt the great need to now pursue, even though rather late in life, my desire to set up an educational institution which would conform to the principles I had been brought up with. In my travels I had visited North-East India and found that in Tripura there was a great need for quality education as well as teaching of values. I found also that there was a core group of young people, whom I could rely upon to take charge of the school and administer it in conformity with Baha'i principles. Thus came into existence the Brilliant Stars School, in the small town of Udaipur, in Tripura. It involved starting from scratch. I was fortunate to get a like-minded partner, who was ready to give back to society and not expect any returns on our capital or on earnings from the school. I got totally involved in the choosing of the land, its purchase, and the construction of the buildings as per the typical houses in the area. Things moved fast, and before we knew it, we had a full-fledged school. It took about five years for the school to become self-sufficient, and till that time, my partner and I, with the help of some generous donors, supported the school. Every year we make two or three visits to the school, to enjoy seeing it grow to be considered the best school in that region. Our alumni are scattered all over India, pursuing different career studies. Going by the principle of being useful to society, we set up an activity in the school for children from Class 5 to Class 10, called the Service Learning Project.

Once a year, these children get together and choose the issue on which they would like to concentrate which affects their society. For example, thre have been projects on Malaria, Swine Flu, Nutrition, Waste Management, and many others. This meant that the children would go on video call to different authorities in India, on the subject, and consult with them, and these projects got documented. The children would make their parents aware of the issues and get their support, and many times change the thinking of the parents. For example, some children used to bring cake and chips for their tea break. After the project on nutrition, the children asked parents for nutritious snacks.

One of the activities that came my way when I turned 80 was to write a book for children on the United Nations Human Rights Declaration. This was due to the fact that people needed to know not only their rights but also their responsibilities as valued citizens of the country. This occupation, I think, has helped me in retaining my memory, and in preventing the degeneration of the brain. The book is being used in some schools, and even as a book in an adult book reading group, where discussions take place on the relevance of each Article of the Declaration.

I believe being active both in mind and body, is very necessary if one does not wish to feel one's old age. Physical exercise and mental exercise are needed simultaneously to maintain the proper balance. It is sad to see people take no interest in life after a certain age and then tend to become a burden on their near and dear ones and on society. I am grateful that I had the opportunity to be of some service to society and I hope that some of these activities will be sustained and prove beneficial to future generations. I thank God for His kindness to me to give me His grace to lead a healthy and, I think, a useful life.

44
In Search of Truth
Dr. Jyotsna Chatterjee

"*The truth will liberate us!*" This old adage always fascinated me. What exactly did it mean? How does truth free us from our shackles? I was to find this out in three events that changed my life completely.

I was brought up in a very conservative Bengali family where my father, the head of the house, took all decisions and my educated mother accepted them without question. However, they had similar opinions regarding the education of their children. Thus, my sisters, my brother and I, were given the same opportunities to complete higher education and secure jobs as principals of schools, an IAS officer and as a college professor. Of course, there was a rider: "see that you do not dishonour the family name".

Three Events that Shaped My Life

The first event that changed my life was marriage. I was fortunate. I married a person who had the same perspective as me and believed that both men and women are equal before God and equal before the Constitution of India. He said to me: "If you want to change the world, you cannot do so by drawing your conclusions from a bird's eye view of the world. You must crawl on the ground and have a snake's eye view of reality." His words rang true and stayed with me and became a guideline for my future actions. Together we walked the path of truth, not only to set ourselves free, but also to try and bring change in the lives of others. We worked as equal partners to ensure social justice in our professions, and in the home.

The second event was the change of my professional life. From being a professor of English Literature in Calcutta University, I established an NGO, Joint Women's Programme (JWP), for the empowerment and education of women and children of marginalised communities. Our work in the JWP was to search for the Truth behind the bondage and violence experienced by women and girls, in every walk of life. I learnt that women and children were more impacted than men by divisions of caste, class, religion, language, education, age, and cultural and customary practices. Also, their marital status made a difference – single, married, divorced, or widowed. This learning opened new vistas for action for change in the violent, violated, and discriminated condition of women in general, in the home and in our society.

The third event was when Dr. V. Mohini Giri ji and Dr. Syeda Hameedji visited me soon after my widowhood and encouraged me to continue my work with renewed strength and vigour in the footsteps of those who had struggled for Justice for Women and the marginalised communities. I continued to gather strength and build relationships in my struggle for truth, realising that the problem of injustice is so vast that to change the situation, the struggle must be carried forward with many partners. Mobilised action at all levels is necessary.

Action for Change

As a Member of the Governing Body of several urban-, rural- and slum-organizations, several special experiences challenged me and taught me how to deal with situations. There were some who held their meetings in air-conditioned rooms and others under the shade of a tree in their courtyard. Each one was struggling to change the existing malnutrition, gender injustice, poverty, and caste/class/ religious discrimination. Each of them, a challenge, a learning, an advice, and a direction towards ways to address situations.

Along with seven National Women's organisations, my colleagues and I addressed the issues of discrimination and violence, and its impact on women and girls. We required changes in the attitude of society regarding the female gender. The demand for several protective laws for women and girls was made to the government. After much struggle and advocacy, the government conceded and prepared new laws, and changed existing old ones to ensure that protection and constitutional justice is provided to women and girls.

A demand made by women's organisations was accepted by the government and the National Commission for Women (NCW) was set up to address issues of discrimination and violence, conduct research and studies on women to prevent violence and promote equality. Under the leadership of Dr. V. Mohini Giri, Chairperson of the NCW at that time, the problems of widows and their status in Indian society became a special focus of attention. Research studies and conferences were organised in various States to understand the impact of religious, cultural, and customary practices on their lives; also, to understand why widows left their hometowns and regions to live in ashrams in holy cities like Varanasi, Mathura, Vrindavan, Haridwar, etc. We found that the majority of these widows were ignorant, uninformed, afraid, and poor. They had internalised their inferior status and were incapable of breaking the existing socio-cultural norms. As a widow from an educated privileged family, I found the condition of widows in general a situation that needed immediate attention for change.

With the help of Dr. V. Mohini Giri, I was able to visit Ma Dham, a widows' home in Vrindavan, Uttar Pradesh, run by the Guild of Service. This gave me the opportunity to interact with inmates, especially Bengali widows, to find out why they had left their own homes, and whether they were pushed out due to family pressure. The widows were afraid to respond, though some revealed that it was difficult for them to continue to live where they were not wanted because of cultural and religious fetters. A few of them had been forced by the family members to leave their homes, and some were even accompanied by male members who left them in ashrams. We found that widows in the Ashram shared a similar pain. They were happy in their togetherness, and thus did not feel the urge to return home. Some Bengali women however, expressed their interest in returning to their hometowns, if they were provided with jobs, for their sustenance, and a place to live.

JWP colleagues, Ms. Amima Mondol, Ms. Sujita Biswas and I, organised a Consultation on "Widows, Neglect and Social Action" in Kolkata. Dr. V. Mohini Giri and NCW were our partners. We invited the West Bengal Ministers of Home, Finance, and Law (who willingly participated) to interact with the representatives of widows, social activists, and NGOs. The West Bengal government responded positively and agreed to rehabilitate Bengali widows in their native towns provided they had the skill to become helpers and teachers in local primary schools and shops. Unfortunately, this did not work as the widows were scared to take up the responsibility. They had been deprived of education, and freedom during their childhood and adolescence, and therefore had no courage, nor the spirit to accept change.

This learning experience forced us to accept the fact that society had continued to neglect women, of whatever category they belonged to, and prevent them from being educated, confident and skilled human beings. They were only considered as homemakers. We were now faced with another dilemma and the knowledge that the denial of education, information, and skill robs women of their free will, their ability to take decisions, and their urge to be participants in the process of social development.

Working with Marginalised Women and Children Provided an Invaluable Foundation

JWP had earlier conducted two short surveys in Karnataka, one of widows in the Bagalur Layout slum, Bengaluru, and the other in the Kolar Gold Fields. In both cases, the widows had not left their hometowns and had found jobs as domestic workers, corporation workers and helpers in the gold mines. Though ostracised from attending religious festivals and marriages, they continued to live in their homes. The other finding was that they belonged to the Dalit and backword communities and were without any training and education, but willing to take up any job for wages. We concluded, that in their communities, religio-cultural factors had a lesser hold on the lives of women. Survival was the deciding factor.

Another study during this period, was again in Karnataka, in two cities and two villages, on "The Status of Single Women" with Dr. Krishna Kumari and other JWP staff, to know whether single women suffered the same fate as widows did, because they had no male support. This study cut across religious and caste lines. Of the women respondents, Hindu women were the least educated, denied freedom, controlled, and depressed. Conditions were slightly better among upper caste women. Muslim women had comparatively a better position, though still controlled and dominated. Christian women had more or less equal opportunities with men to study and procure jobs as doctors, teachers, nurses etc. However, the Indian cultural mindset had pushed all women into becoming second class citizens, denied any status and violated mentally, physically, and emotionally. Our study proved the truth that single women widows, divorced or unmarried, suffered a similar fate in Indian society. Without male support, they were incomplete as human beings, and were regarded rather as evil omens, and witches. The situation varied in degree in relation to their caste, tribe, class, religion, and region they came from. This knowledge strengthened our plan of action to change existing social conditions and attitudes towards single women, whether widowed or unmarried.

JWP discovered that the Devadasi practice in North Karnataka was actually prostitution, with religious sanction. Girl children were dedicated and married to the Goddess Yellamma, on one pretext or the other, and later sexually exploited by priests and landlords. They were also taken to the red-light areas in big metropolitan cities like Mumbai, Kolkata, and Hyderabad, etc. JWP conducted a study led by our colleagues Ms. Asha Ramesh, and Ms. Philomena H. P. who established the extent and spread of the practice, the sexual abuse of girls, and the supply chain for their trafficking from the villages to the red-light areas in metropolitan cities. I proposed a law to ban the Devadasi practice. The Karnataka government enacted the Karnataka Devadasis (Prohibition of Dedication) Act. This was later endorsed by the Central Government. Based on our study on the Devadasis, a film titled *Giddh (The Vulture)*, was made by T. S. Ranga, starring renowned actors (the late) Ms. Smita Patil, (the late) Mr. Om Puri, and Nana Patekar. The film won the Special Jury Award at the National Film Awards festival.

Girls were also disappearing from our project areas, and news reports informed us about increasing trafficking of girls for sexual exploitation. With the support of UNIFEM and some partner organisations, like STOP, SANLAAP, Prajwala, Shakti Vahini and Prayas, we convened a National Consultation and later conducted a study across India, specifically highlighting the problem in metropolitan cities, towns and villages. The study *Trafficking of Women and Girls in India* analysed the problem and recommended to the government the need for changes in the existing law and the policies, to strengthen the prevention of the practice, and the protection and rehabilitation of rescued girls and women. This was followed by another Study and Consultation on *Cross Border Trafficking*.

Ms. Kiran Bedi, formerly the Joint Police Commissioner of Delhi, suggested that I study the conditions of women convicts and detainees in jails across India. With the support of the NCW and my colleague Dr. Jyoti Seth of Chandigarh University we conducted two sample studies (***The situation of Women in the Prisons of Punjab and Chandigarh and Women Prisoners with Children in the Jails of Punjab and Chandigarh.***) Our twosStudies revealed shocking details in the manner in which women convicts and undertrial prisoners were confined and treated by predominantly male officials. This was another angle added to our learning, especially studying about the children below the age of seven, who without any cause had to be confined in these inhuman conditions with their mothers (in accordance with the existing procedures). We recommended better conditions and possibilities for the provision of health needs, education (creches and balwadis), and recreation facilities. The NCW presented these recommendations to the Government for necessary action.

At the request of NHRC and UNICEF, JWP joined hands with India Alliance for Child Rights and Ms. Razia Ismail to understand the National Policy for Children, conduct an All-India study, and pinpoint the reasons for the neglect and violence against children, especially girl children. The cultural practice of child marriage and child labour was studied in detail. Our study of the above two areas recommended that both child labour and child marriage should be abolished. Two laws were passed – *The Child and Adolescent Labour (Prohibition and Regulation) Act* of 1986, which was later amended in 2016 and, *The Prohibition of Child Marriage Act*, 2006", which also was later amended in 2016. Today, despite these laws, the two problems continue because of patriarchy and poverty.

Changes in Personal Laws

Another area that I got involved in, urged by women who came with domestic problems, was the bias in their existing personal laws. Christian women desired equal rights in cases of divorce, as well as in property rights. After several meetings with advocates (Mr. P. M. Bakshi, Late Ms. Kapila Hingorani and Late Ms. Lotika Sarkar) and Church leaders of different denominations, our argument was finally accepted. I was able to convince the then Minister of Law of the Govt. of India, the late Shri Arun Jaitley, to amend Section 10 of the Indian Divorce Act, to ensure that both men and women were given equal grounds for divorce. I also helped Ms. Mary Roy in her endeavour to abolish the existing Travancore and Cochin Succession Act and ensure daughters' rights to property under the Indian Succession Act.

JWP had also taken up the issue of changes in Muslim Personal Laws. These personal laws also perpetuate patriarchal control.

Training Workshops on Gender Justice for Police and Government Personnel

With the Ministry of Women & Children as our partner, we organised police training awareness workshops on Gender Justice. The National Human Rights Commission (NHRC), The National Institute of Criminology and Forensic Science, National Institute of Public Cooperation and Child Development, requested me to become a part of their training and awareness programmes as a Trainer, and the NHRC requested me to organise Police Training programmes in several police training institutions. The first of these was held in Ahmedabad in partnership with the NHRC. My colleague Ms. Anju Grover prepared the slides and helped me in the process. The workshops were helpful for us to examine and, on that basis, to suggest how the police should function in cases of gender violence.

I was open to all organisations who requested JWP to partner with them in the search for equal justice for women. Several organisations, NGOs, corporates, hotel industry, universities, colleges, and departments of the Government of India, requested me to organise training workshops on Gender Justice and specifically on sexual harassment in the workplace.

To make it possible to inform organisations of various kinds and the general public on what sexual harassment in the workplace means, JWP in partnership with The Asia Foundation, New Delhi, and the Indian National Bar Association, organised a training workshop on *The Sexual Harassment at the Workplace (Prevention, Protection and Redressal) Act*, 2013. This training programme gave us closer understanding of the functioning of that Act. It also enabled us to be associated with legal luminaries who expressed their opinion that such workshops are essential for awareness-generation and action.

Mera Sahara – Education cum Protection Centre for Children and Women

In December 2006, the newspapers reported an incident of sexual abuse, kidnapping, and massacre of several children in Nithari Village, in Noida, Uttar Pradesh. The village is inhabited by migrant labour from various parts of India, engaged in construction work, corporation labour, and domestic work. Some are rickshaw pullers, ragpickers, etc. Since both parents work, the children were roaming the streets and falling prey to antisocial elements. Rape, sale, and trafficking were rampant. JWP's survey conducted here revealed the absence of schools, balwadis, and ICDS programmes, that we demanded from the U. P. Government. I started a Protection-cum-Learning Centre called JWP 'Mera Sahara', along with my colleagues, Ms. Vijay Bala, Ms. Padmini Kumar, and Ms. Bimla Patni. Local donations from friends made this possible. We sensitised the parents to prevent violence and enable JWP to create a safe and happy place for their children. Mera Sahara and its local watchdog group of parents encouraged us to prevent child marriage, child labour, trafficking, and kidnapping. So far, we have been able to help over 1,500 children to get admission to mainstream schools after completing Class V at our Centre. Adult education and skill training for community women and girls is also undertaken here. The USHA Silai School initiative provides training in tailoring and the possibility of economic empowerment to women and girls, by providing free sewing machines, after their successful training. We need to continue to raise funds for the continuity of this initiative which has prevented gender violence to a large extent by making women economically more self-sufficient.

Working with War Widows: **Veer Naries**

Dr. V. Mohini Giri gave me the opportunity to be a consultant to the War Widows Association (WWA), in New Delhi. As I worked with them, organising training programmes and meetings with war widows in different areas, I realised that the same problems of caste, class, customs, lack of education, authority, and denial of equal rights affected them as well, though varying in degree. In one case the widow of a martyred Jawan with two daughters was murdered by family members who hoped to claim the financial benefits provided to her by the Government of India. Their reason was that since the Jawan was their son, the compensation on his death should go to his parents and brothers and not his wife. This is another proof of the patriarchal control on women's lives and property. With both parents' dead the two little daughters had no support, and the WWA took up the matter. The two girls were provided all support for their education and training and are now being enabled to find employment.

To ensure that all War Widows received their benefits as planned by the government, I helped the late Ms. Dolly Singh, the former President of WWA, and Ms. Prema Kala of WWA, to organise a Consultation on *National Policy for the Rehabilitation and Welfare of Widows of War and Armed Conflict*. The then Defence Minister, Shri A. K. Anthony and several government officials participated in the same. Dr. V. Mohini Giri was the Chairperson of the Consultation. The widows of Kargil and other wars, participated in the Consultation and shared their needs and grievances regarding the disbursal of benefits from the concerned State departments. Several war widows were unaware of the government schemes, especially those who lived in far-flung villages and were therefore deprived of all their benefits. For WWA, this was additional understanding of the status of widows and the need for intervention where justice was denied.

Economic Empowerment – A Crucial Need

There was need to ensure that women be trained and skilled to be economically empowered so that they did not have to depend solely on the male family members. JWP introduced various skill training and adult education programmes for women, to enable them to find jobs with suitable wages. This made them economically empowered, capable, and confident enough to take up jobs. The Government and several other NGOs have created schemes and programmes for skill training and employment with suitable wages. They have also emphasised the need for equal wages for women. Educational institutions, the corporate, government departments, including the defence sector, are now employing women, and finding women to be at par with men in their performance.

Women's Right to Decision Making

Basing our work on the results of the study on the *Status of Women in India* by the late Dr. Veena Majumdar, we accepted that Gender, Caste and Cultural differences dominate the lives of all people and make it impossible for women to participate in decision making in the home and in larger society. State Assemblies and Parliament also deny them this right. Our demand has been "**Give us at least 33%, if not 50%** reservation of seats in Sate Assemblies and Parliament", so that women's issues can be discussed by them in the political arena, and suitable legislation and policies for their citizens' rights and dignity can be addressed by their participation. Unfortunately, the same patriarchal mindset as explained above has prevented successive Governments from implementing this demand, even today.

The Truth Shall Set You Free – The Need for Change

Despite protective laws, policies, and schemes, there has been little change in the mindset of society at large. The continuing number of rapes, harassment, murder, domestic violence, sale, and torture has increased women's fear of pursuing their personal interests. Today, even though many women have the opportunity of employment and are informed about the laws and policies for their protection, they are still afraid to break the chains of bondage. Men and women continue to be controlled by the old ***sanskaar*** rather than by laws and policies framed under the Constitution of India.

Today our hope lies with the young citizens of India, who are learning to break away from existing practices and are questioning patriarchy and other unequal social norms. Our job now is to ensure that we support and strengthen them and continue with them in the struggle and demand for Equality before Law and Equal Protection of the Law.

Age Has Been No Factor

I have often been asked the question, "Now that you are 81 years old, what is your feeling regarding your work and your age?" This question I have not been able to answer, as I still continue to be involved in work, conducting training and participating in discussions and related action, (except when my body is aching all over!). I still continue to intervene without fear and constraint. What has driven me and given me the energy to continue in my search and necessary action, is my belief that if conditions are unjust and wrong, they must be attended to. I am not alone in this: several of my friends and partners in the struggle for change, close to my age, have grown gracefully and youthfully along with me. **We are still young!**

Several years of experience have given us a clearer understanding of how to address a concern in a better way. Unfortunately, equality, justice and a violence-free world for all are eluding us. Perhaps we have not fully understood the strength of the existing socio-cultural fabric that envelops us, and our world. The new generation of informed and sensitive citizens will take forward what we have begun and fulfil the goal that we have striven for, with greater energy.

Still More Miles to Go

As I dealt with each situation and planned interventions and actions together with others, a world of fellowship and joint action opened up before me, making possible new ideas, actions, and dialogues across all political ideologies. A large number of groups of women and men, who believed in the Constitutional guarantees joined us, to make several changes in laws, policies, schemes and practices, thus gradually improving the conditions of all marginalised communities, in order to improve the status of women who are a part of each caste, class, ethnicity and religion. This struggle for justice that we have embarked on together is not over and must continue to be strengthened until justice and peace is established in our homes, in our society, in our country, and in the World.

As the famous poet **Robert Frost** wrote:

The woods are lovely, dark and deep.
But I have promises to keep,
And miles to go before I sleep,
And miles to go before I sleep.

45
Growing Old Gracefully
Kalpakam Yechury

What a lovely concept.

It is lovely to think we are the lucky people to be in this group. How we grew, we really did not realise. Suddenly children celebrated our 80th birthday! Oh God, I am 80, I felt. No health problems to remind me of my age, going to my NGO regularly, driving my car as usual. So I didn't bother about the numbers as they were increasing.

Luckily I am working in a group that had ladies of the same mentality so there was no question of discussing age or habits or changes in the mind or body. You have to be lucky in many ways to grow gracefully. Our inheritance is the first advantage – coming from a family with longevity, so we imbibed the mentality of not thinking of age. We automatically continue to live comfortably without realising we are growing old. Of course, we are growing old, but the pace of living has not changed for us. At 80, I wanted to renew my car driving licence. At at that point, there were no rules to give licences to those over 80 years. The officer told me, "Madam at your age, you should have the luxury of a driver." I told him that I was nervous if someone drove me and I was more comfortable driving myself. I could have driven up to 85, but then thinking of others' safety I stopped driving.

Habits make us what we are. Even here luck comes in, whichever country we lived in or in whatever situations, we were able to follow our own habits, and eat whatever we are accustomed to. Being a vegetarian, I eat only vegetables and pulses as simple food. Curds were a must wherever we were, whatever the weather was, and luckily it suited me.

Our attitude towards life is the same – ups and downs are always there, but a positive attitude to deal with problems makes everything a pleasure. I was lucky that I inherited the attitude that I could pass through life without many changes.

Above all this is my philosophy of life, the Indian thought of life and Karma theory:

Karmanyeshuvadhikaraste
Maphaleshu kadachana

I am responsible for my actions not for the fruits. I will do whatever He had ordained me to do. Maybe this is the best way of living life which makes us forget age and live in the actions of the present.

I thank God that I have lived the right way and give the credit to God.

46
Ageing Positively, Productively, and Gracefully
Asha Das

When I was asked to write on this topic, I wondered whether there was any other way to age. I don't remember taking a conscious decision to grow older – positively, productively, gracefully – but as I reflect back on the past 20 years, I seem to have done so. My years as a senior citizen have been as fulfilling and joyful, as the six decades before. With humility, and with the intention of sharing what has contributed to my happiness over the years, I agreed to write this piece.

Our life as a senior citizen begins at 60 according to popular definition. I remember, very clearly, as I approached that magic number. As a civil servant for 38 years, work had been an integral part of my adult life – and one fine day, long before I was physically, mentally or emotionally ready for it – it was coming to an abrupt end. The truth is, even as I worried occasionally about a day there would be no office to go to, I was never apprehensive about the transition from being a full-time civil servant to a retired one. I was, in fact, quite excited about all the things I had hoped to have time to do 'some day'. And now, 'some day' was finally here with all the freedom one could ask for.

The reason for this, perhaps, was that to me ageing was always clearly on the horizon – and I expected it to be like other previous phases of life where changes came along, and slipped gently into the way I lived. Ageing felt natural and inevitable, unless of course, if life is cut short for reasons beyond our control. Our transition from childhood to youth, and adulthood are seldom accompanied by fear – in fact, there is often excitement about moving to the next phase. As we grow from childhood to youth, we move from a life dependent on nurturing, care and protectiveness, to higher studies sometimes away from home, choosing a career, and becoming independent, self-reliant and confident. Our expectations, aspirations, duties, and responsibilities also change significantly, as we advance in our careers and personal lives, and start families. We learn to balance our duties, and responsibilities not only towards family and work, but also towards wider relationships, and social and other commitments that give us happiness and satisfaction in life.

Not to say that I wasn't conscious of the doubts, fears and anxieties that are such an integral part of each phase and transition. Failures, difficulties and bereavements are a part of each of our lives, as are successes, expanding families, and joys. Over time, we learn to look at our life as a whole, with a sense of fulfilment. And therefore I wonder why we look at the transition to 'senior citizenship' with more fear than excitement? Is it because we get so used to a disciplined and busy life with responsibilities on both the home and work front that the sudden loss of assigned work and responsibilities distresses us? Is it because we withdraw and then feel that life is coming to an end? Or is it because we don't accept our old age as a progressive part of our life and feel disheartened not only at the loss of occupation but also at the imminent change in our environment and lifestyle? Personally, I felt it would be a different life – not worse – and was nervously excited about the freedom and the opportunity to do several things I had always wanted to, without the constraints of my working life.

It was November the 1st, 2001. My first day of retirement. I had not planned my future, but I had many choices in front of me – I could enjoy a leisurely morning, potter about in the garden, start reading from the stack of unread books, visit parents, children, siblings, friends, go and see new and interesting places and even find new things to do. Though I was excited about each of these options and indulged myself in the first few months - leisurely doing what I wanted to- to my surprise, I found myself wondering how I could get involved with 'meaningful activities' that would help me to continue being useful and productive. I had enough to think about. I had to start sorting the house to enable my move to my new home. I was also concerned about not having any administrative support as I tried settling into a new life, not having the government machinery to help me get through the day. I realised I was used to the services of efficient personal staff in my many years of service. Clearly, this wasn't going to be a straightforward and easy transition – and it was up to me to make the most of it. There was only one thing I was sure of – I had always adapted very quickly to new situations in my life and this was going to be yet another of those experiences. My inherent approach to life (now referred to as a 'positive approach'!) and capacity to accept changes happily, I knew would see me through without distress or agony. I knew this would be another experience and the beginning of a new phase that I would look back at with the quiet satisfaction of a life well-lived.

As I reflect on my attitude, I realise I had the huge advantage of exemplary role models within the family. I was fortunate to have been brought up in a family where my parents looked after not only six of their own children but also my grandparents, uncles and aunts, their families, and many more. My parents had an open and welcoming house for close as well as distant relatives. They always reached out to people in need of support, despite their very limited resources. They valued and maintained relationships and this seemed to give them a great sense of contentment. My father was a civil servant, but had no savings when he retired at age 58. Having been an upright and honest officer, he knew trying for a job with Government was not a likely future option. He decided to do what he loved most. He had spent his life giving each one of his children the best education, and had guided almost all his siblings and friends' children. He was also very conscious of the fact that Madhya Pradesh had a very poor track record of success in the All India Services – and decided to commit his retired life to coaching young people to join the civil services. He started offering classes in Bhopal, where he and my mother settled, and taught with dedication till he was 93 years old! His smooth transition from an high ranking Administrator to a teacher without any help (he taught what he could as he did not want to run his Centre on commercial lines), his commitment to the youth of Madhya Pradesh, the contentment from helping more than 200 boys and girls join the services was exemplary and inspirational. He enjoyed his retirement years, as much as his working years, if not more, devoting his life to the family and utilising his knowledge and experience in - as they say - 'paying it forward'.

My mother, too, played a hugely important role in shaping my attitude to life. From the very beginning she ensured that we learnt to look after our own and our family's basic needs. We were made conscious from a very early age that all the perks and facilities we enjoyed in our home thanks to our father's position were bonuses – we should never become entitled to them. She firmly believed in girls being economically independent and therefore ensured that all five of us sisters finished our education and chose our own careers before we thought of our marriages. She taught us values that helped us face adversities and accept changes with the equanimity and fortitude so essential for happiness.

Armed with this legacy, I looked at myself on retirement as a person free from the disciplined and planned daily schedule of a working woman. I met friends, specially my women friends with whom I previously was unable to spend time, and enjoyed renewing and rebuilding those bonds. I loved the freedom of unplanned meetings with friends and relatives and realised that renewed contacts often gave me an opportunity to be helpful, which always added meaning to my life.

I was fortunate that my friends and associates of working years kept in touch and even offered opportunities for short term assignments that related to the social sectors I had worked in. Soon after I had settled into my new house, I was offered an assignment with UNIFEM to identify Ministries that could play an important role in managing drug abuse and help build their strategies and programmes. It was a hugely uplifting and liberating experience. Used to staff support through my career, I was apprehensive about managing the research and data collection required for a high-quality report by myself, not to mention the lack of practice in the use of a computer and typing! However, I was determined to do the work on my own without the help of a stenographer (had to fight with my kids for not hiring one!) – and with some help from UNIFEM staff, I was able to prepare the reports myself. This experience did wonders for me – and the only cost was an attack of spondylosis!

Once I began working independently, other projects flowed in. All of these were in sectors that I was familiar with and kept me partially engaged and occupied in the first few years after retirement. I enjoyed discovering issues from a perspective 'outside the government', and also the opportunity to study the programmes and functions of different departments that I hadn't worked in earlier. To see my experience remain valuable, both at the central and state government levels, added to my sense of satisfaction.

In 2005, I was appointed Member Secretary of the National Commission for Religious and Linguistic Minorities for a period of two years by the Ministry of Social Justice and Empowerment. This assignment gave me an opportunity to visit all the States and meet political and administrative heads, NGOs, religious heads, minority community organizations, linguistic minorities, and their representatives. The Report required detailed study about sensitive and complicated issues such as demand by Christian and other converts for the status of SC and STs, grant of reservation in services and educational institutions to minority communities etc. Once again, I found myself learning new things and perspectives and recognised that retirement and senior citizen status certainly did not mean less excitement or purpose.

While these intermittent opportunities were welcome and helped with the transition, what has sustained me in the last 20 years since retirement have been activities, work and a way of livng that I chose.

While in service in 1993-94, I had renewed my association with my college friends. I made time to attend the first couple of meetings despite a gruelling work schedule. But some of us with demanding careers, suggested that, as alumnae of the prestigious Isabella Thoburn College, we should meet to have fun, but also do some substantive work. We decided to register ourselves as a Society and start a school. The SOF (Social Outreach Foundation School) which started in two rooms of DPS, Noida, in 1995, for children from slums, has now been running for 25 years as a primary school in a rented building and is supporting 300 students. We added support for higher secondary education, and for employment-oriented skill development programmes.

Since retirement I have been actively involved in its running. I feel satisfied and proud when I see many of our children join good colleges, take professional degrees and establish themselves as teachers, chartered accountants, obtain scholarships to go abroad and study etc. Today, many of our alumni come back to school to say they want to help other children like themselves. The circle of life and 'paying it forward' continues unabated.

Mohini Giri and I had earlier had the opportunity to work together (in 1997-98) – she as Chairman of the National Commission for Women, and I as Secretary of the Ministry of Woman and Child Development. We had studied the problems of widows in Vrindavan, and conceived a plan to start a home for them. Subsequently Mrs Giri raised funds to construct a home to house 200 widows. I am associated with the home and Guild of Service activities and programmes for the economic empowerment of women through training and skill development. It has been a rewarding experience and a source of joy over the years to continue to be usefully engaged in improving the lives of needy women. I have also been associated with Guild in planning and development of programmes for children affected by terrorism in Jammu and Kashmir.

Besides the Guild of Service, I am associated with several other NGOs – the Amar Jyoti Foundation and the Akshay Pratishthan which are engaged in providing services and training to the differently-abled.

My interest and commitment for the care, protection and welfare of children, women and the elderly has continued after retirement. The lack of trained workers to provide care and support services to the aged living on their own had caused me a great deal of anxiety ever since I drew up the policy for the Aged as Secretary for Social Justice and Empowerment. The fact that Govt policies and programmes looked after the destitute women and elderly only, and for destitute and orphaned children till the age of age of 18, and gave skeletal after-care for them until they turned 21, always troubled me. I had registered a society in 1985 to start some welfare programmes. When I was appointed as Joint Secretary in 1986 in the Ministry responsible for the above segments, I chose to let the Society remain dormant.

However when I was free to pursue what I liked and wanted to, I realized that one's capacity to learn and continue to be productively useful to the needy does not come to an end at age 60 or thereafter. One can continue to contribute effectively to the well being of others.

I knew that we urgently needed trained personnel to provide services to the elderly living on their own and capable of paying for these services - healthy older people with normal ageing problems. On retirement, I developed a program to train young women for providing home-based services tothe elderly. While basic medical care and knowledge of age-related medical needs were included, emphasis was on the physical, nutritional, psychological, emotional and safety needs of the elderly. We conducted several courses over 2-3 years in Delhi and Bhopal.

I was able to get the assistance of experts and professionals from medical and nursing Institutes, Lady Irwin College, Helpage India, and many others. It was an enriching experience and the curriculum we developed was later launched by several others. It felt good that something I had started was going to make a difference in a much larger sphere.

I also worked with the Aurobindo Ashram to conduct a five-day course to discuss the issues of child care with rural women, with a view to addressing the rising delinquency among children when they are left unsupervised. This is a program I am still interested in pursuing!

Apart from the above I have spent time visiting family and friends, and travelling to new places with them, which keeps me entertained.

I have now had 20 years of retired life. It has been different from my younger days – but equally enriching, and with the good fortune of not having any regrets. While each one of us has a unique life, situation, personality and expectations, there may be some recipes from my life that might have a relevance to others. Three overarching principles have guided my life and I will try my best to describe them here.

First, Be helpful.

We can worry that as we get older we don't have the power or the influence that we had in our earlier days and therefore feel less relevant and useful. I have found that we need to change the way we think and can help. Through all these years I have continued to feel relevant and productive. I have consciously invested my time and energy in building and strengthening relationships. I enjoy meeting and spending time with people I am fond of – good friends and family keep us away from loneliness, and help us keep healthy and happy. Doing things together gives joy, and helping each other through difficulties keeps you feeling relevant. I feel I have continued to contribute positively to others - my children's friends and colleagues, my friends and relatives, and many others. In doing so I have used my connections and the access my position and friendships during working life have given me, very freely. Being helpful to the extent you can and contributing tangibly to the extent you can is the key to being positively engaged. So we don't need to shy away from being helpful. Our power and capacity to help doesn't end at 60.

Secondly, Volunteer Your Time.

At 60, we are physically, mentally, emotionally and psychologically fit. Neither of these changes overnight. My association with NGOs and my desire to continue to contribute to improve and upgrade the lives of needy children, women and the marginalised sections of society has helped me to keep myself engaged comfortably and meaningfully. My association with organisations like the Aurobindo Ashram and Samarth – an organisation providing valuable and much needed support services to the economically independent aged – gives me opportunity both to contribute productively and extend help to those who need it. Voluntary work for a good cause, while helping you to be useful, also gives you a sense of purpose.

Thirdly, Take Ggrowing Older in Your Stride!

Growing old is a natural phenomenon of life. Embracing apprehensions about ageing – loss of regular work and profession, the supporting staff, perks and facilities, the power and access I enjoyed for extending help and services, and of course the fear of age-related health issues cropping up as a part of life ahead - have all helped me in adopting a positive approach to life.

As a single person, with my children having completed their education and settled in their own lives, I felt free to lead my own life. Being confident and aware that I wanted to lead an independent life as long as possible, I did want to have enough time for children, as and when they were free, to be with them and also be able to help them whenever they needed it. I have led a happy and fulfilling life pursuing voluntary and other work, spending time with friends and relatives, visiting places with friends and family within the country and outside, visiting and looking after my parents while they were here, happily helping those who needed it to the extent I could. I try to strike a balance in things I want to do and enjoy doing, sharing and hopefully distributing happiness and living positively, even as I am ageing.

The ageing phase in life is when, while enjoying children, grandchildren, friends and relatives, you have time to pursue things left undone in the preceding decades happily.

47

AGEING GRACEFULLY

SUNANDA SINGHANIA

The very thought of sharing experiences on ageing gracefully triggers a host of emotions, as we pause and reflect on the journey of life. The world that we knew in our childhood has changed in every aspect, and will continue to do so. How does one age gracefully? Perhaps there is no single answer.

Times are bound to change, as change is a constant. What is of essence is our ability to adapt to, as well as embrace, that change. The values imbibed in childhood play a major role in this. Hailing from a business family and marrying into one was a major milestone. It is my privilege and the blessings of the Almighty to have as my life partner Dr. Raghupati Singhania. We have walked together hand in hand over the years as friends and companions. We have learnt from each other.

Material wealth beyond a point holds limited value and it is inner satisfaction that really matters and indeed helps. With this approach, age as they say is just a number and it is all in the mind. One aspect which stands out very clearly is that our physical and mental disposition shapes our lives. This is very evident when we look around us and realise that happiness and contentment, as they both come from within, play a major role in ageing gracerully.

Not only should one not do anything for the sake of doing it, but if we do it as a passion and not as a task, any achievement therein becomes self-motivating. Thus not only are we happily engaged but as we keep working towards our goals, we discover newer challenges.

One of my initial pursuits was Indian classical dance, and I was happy that my dedication was recognized by being awarded a Gold Medal. Being a student of Indian classical vocal music led to a greater appreciation of music. Both these pursuits have enabled me to channel energies and remain agile in every aspect over the years. This demonstrates the importance of having a hobby which becomes a pursuit and a passion.

When one enjoys the beauty of flowers in diverse forms with the changes of season, when a bloom comes only for a few days, then we realize that there is a greater force that has created nature. Maintaining a garden has a special place in my heart and has always been very fascinating. Needless to say, when you get accolades for pursuing your hobby it is a great encouragement. Looking back, I feel gratified that my dedication to gardening resulted in our garden in Delhi getting the first prize for a number of years. Every time I travel in India and abroad, visiting gardens and learning about plants and flowers is a must on my itinerary.

Visiting places in India and the world is a must for me. This can be for work, or just for a complete break from the daily routine. This lets me refresh, renew, and re-energise. The family business instincts and genes were bound to show up somewhere. So the fondness for travelling translated itself into a fully-fledged travel agency, which takes up some of my time.

No man is an island, and we all have various social circles and events, starting with family, friends, colleagues, business associates, business functions, festivals, and other platforms. One can choose to live in isolation or lead an active social life. While it is not possible to be everywhere, we must try to stay connected to the extent possible and lead a balanced social life. The very fact that one readies oneself for an occasion or an interaction becomes a driving force. Not only social circles, but public events, musical recitals, theatres and unforgettable movies, whether at home or at a cineplex, show us the diversity of life and also expose us to wider experiences from which we can learn a lot.

The ethos of Indian culture of sharing and giving, irrespective of socio-economic status, is very deep rooted in our family. We believe in the thought "*Vasudhaiva Kutumbakam*". We must give back to society as much as our resources permit. Giving back does not mean just monetary support but going out and helping the less-privileged or creating platforms and facilities which can benefit society. It is a very fulfilling process.

We were able to establish South-East Asia's first, super specialty hospital for digestive diseases, which went to become a leading multi-speciality hospital of Delhi, known as the Pushpawati Singhania Hospital & Research Institute – PSRI Hospital. I have been involved in this Institute ever since its inception. It gives me great satisfaction to be able to provide healthcare to society at large. I am proud that we do so in a very ethical manner.

So how has all this been possible?

First of all, we must understand that ageing is inevitable. How we cope with it is a matter of our aptitude, attitude, and application towards this fact of life. This begins with an understanding of self, our thoughts, our values, and our purpose in life. As we progress in years, our needs change. Though one may state that basic needs remain the same at any stage – food, shelter, and safety - the needs change from physiological to psychological, and then to self fulfilment. If we recognise these well in time, we can cope with the process of ageing.

In my earlier years perhaps it would have been my endeavor to pursue new hobbies and establish new ventures; but over a period of time the greater focus is on qualitative improvements, and sustaining existing pursuits rather than just quantitative growth.

Some treasures that help us to age gracefully:

- **Good Physique:** One can avoid physical dependence by exercising regularly. Over a period of time Yoga helps. Good sleep is a very vital factor. Drinking lots of water is essential.
- **Eating Right:** Healthy and traditional foods are always recommended, and generations have not been able to find

fault with those. However, medical guidance, depending on health condition, should be adhered to. We must remember nutritional needs change as one ages.

- **Attitude:** Be positive for the sake of your own mental and emotional health.
- **Attachment:** We must practice detachment, and let go where required.
- **Moderation:** Moderation in everything we do is extremely important.
- **Spiritual:** Practice mindfulness, which is acceptance and living in the moment. Mindfulness enables one to focus, reduces stress, controls emotions. One can meditate, and read scriptures which tell us the real meaning of life.

It was thanks to my father that in my early years, I was initiated by a spiritual Guru. This has been a great blessing in my life. It has taught me to stay calm at all times, more so in times of stress. It has been a great strength to me. This emanates from an unquestionable faith and belief in the Creator.

A challenge that comes with ageing is a feeling of irrelevance which leads to larger problems. It should be remembered that life has not come to a halt. There are many ways one can contribute to society, starting with neighborhood. Let youngsters know you are available to them to teach a skill, to mentor, or to be a guide. Impart knowledge wherever possible. But never be judgemental.

For the self, we must try to remember that any skill or hobby or educational course, or language one may have wanted to learn or do in busier days, and could not, it is never too late to learn something new.

I would like to say that it is important to pursue some hobby or a cause in life to keep busy and make life meaningful. Whatever one chooses must be done with full commitment and passion. This will certainly be highly satisfying, and success is bound to follow. As somebody had said: "Reboot, Reinvent, Rewire".

We need to remember, that we need not regret getting older – it is a privilege denied to many.

I look back with great satisfaction at the years gone by. Sometimes I wonder what I could have done better. But I have no regrets, and rather than ruminating about the past I would prefer to look forward to the years that the Almighty may bestow on me and enjoy life as it comes.

In conclusion, I would like to quote Robert Frost, as these line sum up my mind set beautifully:

"***The woods are lovely, dark and deep,***
but I have promises to keep, and miles to go before I sleep".

48
Ageing
Dr. Lalit Bhasin

Age is a number, but ageing is a process. Ageing is defined in the dictionaries as a state of maturity or ripeness.

In my profession, which is law, age or ageing signifies more and more maturity, brilliance, creation of wealth of knowledge, coupled with unique experience and expertise. After Mr. Ram Jethmalani, one of the legends in the field of law reached the age of 85 he told his colleagues and juniors that although he was waiting in the Departure Lounge of life it did not mean that he would stop practising law. He remained as active as any young lawyer and retained his full mental faculties till he left the Departure Lounge in his mid-nineties to board the flight to eternity. A friend of one of the greatest living lawyers of our country asked Fali Nariman, who is in his early nineties as to when he would retire from law practice. The response which Fali gave is acknowledged as a tribute to the legal profession of the country. Fali said, "My friend, in India, we lawyers do not retire – we just drop dead in harness".

We as lawyers remain active and agile till.... In fact, there is no ageing involved and, if at all it is, ageing makes one much better, more sophisticated, and more learned in the discharge of one's duties to the client.

It is a sad state of affairs that our judges of the higher courts have to retire at a comparatively young age before the so-called ageing process starts. High Court judges retire at the age of 62, and Supreme Court judges retire at the age of 65. This is the age when their knowledge, their brilliance and understanding of law is getting more mature. This vast reservoir of talent and brilliance is lost to the country, after their retirement. Some serious thought needs to be given by the people in power that these gems, representing Indian judiciary, should be made to shine much longer instead of being thrown into oblivion.

Sir Jamshedji Kanga in a Foreword to the First Edition of 'Kanga and Palkhivala on Income Tax' wrote: "The riders in a race do not stop short when they reach the goal. There is a little finishing canter before coming to a standstill. There is time to hear the kind voice of friends and to say to oneself, 'The work is done'. But just as one says that, the answer comes: "The race is over, but the work is never done while the power to work remains. The canter that brings you to a standstill need not be only coming to rest. It cannot be while you still live. For to live is to function. That is all there is in living."

F. S. Nariman in his autobiography, "*Before Memory Fades...*" refers to the Principal of Bishop Cotton School where Fali was a student during 1942-43. Each year the Principal bade farewell to his students who passed out of school with the dismal words 'My boys I wish you all a life full of difficulties'. Everyone would think that it was a cruel thing to say. However, after eighty two years of experience in another school – the hard school of life – I am convinced that his words had the merit of wisdom. When you meet with difficulties early in life, the way in which you confront and overcome helps to build your character.

The difficult period for me started when I was eight years old when the Partition of India took place and suddenly, from a comfortable style of living, getting education in the Presentation Convent School in Rawalpindi and owning a car, which was definitely a status symbol at that point of time, we became refugees. My father, late Mr. Tilak Raj Bhasin had a flourishing law practice in Rawalpindi and my mother, late Mrs. Shakuntala Bhasin had ensured the best possible upbringing for my siblings (my twin sisters Rajni and Sajni – five years old, and my brother Suneel Bhasin born in 1946). We were uprooted from hearth and home, and after short stays in Srinagar and Jammu where my maternal grandfather used to live, we finally landed in New Delhi. This was the turning point in our lives and the period of struggle had already started.

Looking back, one is flooded with memories of hardships, discomforts and uncertainties. At the same time, one remembers with great fondness and gratitude the sacrifices made by my parents to provide us with whatever comfort they could provide, without in any way compromising on our educational needs and our diet. Children tend to forget the role played by the parents in bringing them up and enabling them to be good citizens. There can be no substitute for 'family' and particularly the parents. It is only when one looks back that one realizes the sacrifice and role of the parents in bringing up the children. I completed my school education and passed the Higher Secondary examination with flying colours. I was able to get admission in the prestigious Hindu College, Delhi, thanks to the efforts of my parents and also possibly because of my good marks.

The hallmark of a great institution is whether after more than sixty years you can still remember with gratitude those who taught you. My student life in Hindu College became a great pillar of strength for me in my later life mainly because of the brilliance of my teachers and the affection they showered on me. I have nostalgic memories of Hindu College as an institution. This is where way back in 1958 my leadership aptitude came to the fore as I was elected as the Prime Minister of the College Parliament – the highest position a student could achieve in College.

I have tried in my own small way to help and assist Hindu College even after I became a successful lawyer. I have held the position of being the President of Old Students' Association of Hindu College for nearly twenty years. One should always not only remember with gratitude the role which educational institutions have played in one's life, but also to keep bonding with the institutions. This feeling becomes an inspiration for one's own self, that one is giving back in whatever measure one can.

I completed my graduation in 1962 and started law practice in the month of September 1962. For me, my father was a role model. He was one of the most hardworking lawyers I have ever come across and he enjoyed drafting petitions in his own hand as one did not have good and efficient stenographers at that time and in any case my father used to burn the midnight oil and work late till the wee hours. He was brilliant in the court as well. He was a great source of strength for me while he was practicing in Delhi. He later on shifted to Jammu and Kashmir where he was representing ousted leaders like Sheikh Abdullah and Bakshi Ghulam Mohammad. I was virtually on my own from early years of my law practice.

I was married to my Hindu College soul mate Madhu in 1961. Between the years 1963 and 69 my early marriage and birth of my daughters, Sonia, Divvya, Priya and Shilpa ensured that I put in my best as I had a family to support. My wife Madhu who belonged to an extremely well-to-do Marwari family adjusted very well to the low middle class standard of living that we had. My wife Madhu died of lung cancer in 1991. We have four loving daughters and doting sons-in-law and most affectionate and caring grandchildren. My profession gave me my second wife Nina Gupta who had joined my firm in 1979. We got married in 1995 and are blessed with an adoring son Aditya. As in the case of one's parents there is no substitute for the family. I love my entire family and it remains the greatest source of strength to me particularly at this age.

I have held many positions in the profession, in the statutory bodies and in the corporate world. I am not going into the positions that I have held till 1992 when I had completed thirty years in the profession and had been elected as Secretary General of the International Bar Association for the Asia Pacific Region. I was nominated as the Secretary for the Union Internationale des Avocats (Asian Region). I had already held the position of Chairman of Delhi Bar Council. I was sitting on the Board of Directors of the East India Hotels (Oberoi Group), Godfrey

Phillips India Limited, Reliance Petrochemicals Limited, and many other well-known corporate bodies. I became the General Secretary of the Bar Association of India with Mr. Fali Nariman as the President till the year 2010, when I was elevated as the Vice President of the Association and finally as the President of this apex body of the legal profession from 2016 till 2020. During this period, I was also nominated by the Government of India as the Chairman of Films Certification Appellate Tribunal. I have been the President of the Society of Indian Law Firms since its inception in the year 2000. I was the only Indian lawyer to be given the unique honour of Honorary Membership of the International Bar Association way back in 1994 in Melbourne, Australia. During this period, I have received many awards from various organisations, professional bodies and the government including the Award given by the Hon'ble Prime Minister Atal Bihari Vajpayee in the year 2002 for my services to the legal profession, and by the President of India Shrimati Pratibha Patil for maintaining the highest standards in the legal profession in the year 2009.

During this process of what is commonly described as ageing I have learnt a lot and have striven to give something back to society and to the profession. Fruitful and productive ageing can only be achieved if one has the will to keep on working and to share the philosophy of your success with others so that they can emulate you when the ageing process starts.

At 81-plus, what sustains me are:

- The chances and joy of winning a complicated case. This joy should remain, because in India we lawyers prefer to die with our boots on.
- The kindness and affection of my colleagues at the Bar whose company I greatly value and enjoy.
- It is always a good practice to sit in the court during your spare time waiting for your case to be called out, and to listen and to learn regarding the proceedings in other matters.

At this age, one should not think of one's professional future. Professional future has been secured by your achievements in the past.

One should keep on finding ways and means to give back to society.

Live and enjoy the life with the family and…

… keep working.

Section III
About the Authors

Mani Shankar Aiyar is an Indian politician and former career civil servant, diplomat, writer, and acclaimed speaker: As a member of the Indian National Congress Party, he was a nominated member of parliament from Rajya Sabha, and represented the Mayiladuthurai constituency of Tamil Nadu in the 10th Lok Sabha, in the 13th Lok Sabha, and in the 14th Lok Sabha. He is a special invitee to the Congress Working Committee, and was Chairman of both the party's Political Training Department and its Department of Policy Planning and Coordination. A well-known political columnist, his books include *Pakistan Papers* and *Remembering Rajiv*, and he edited the four-volume *Rajiv Gandhi's India*. He is especially interested in grassroots democracy, in Indian foreign policy particularly with respect to India's neighbouring countries, West Asia and nuclear disarmament.

Subhashini Ali: grass roots activist, feminist, human rights activist, joined the Communist Party of India (Marxist), worked in trade unions in Kanpur and was active in the joint women's Anti-Price Rise movement and then in the movement for the restoration of democracy during the Emergency of 1975-77. She was a delegate to the founding conference of the All India Democratic Womens Association (AIDWA) and was elected to the Central Executive Committee of the largest women's organisation in India with membership of over 15,000,000. AIDWA has been regularly organising movements and struggles at the local, state and national levels on every kind of issue involving women, their rights and against their oppression. She was elected to Parliament in 1989 from Kanpur as a CPI(M) candidate. As the member of the National Commission for Women she initiated a study on the impact of the New Economic Policies on the Public Distribution System. She led the 9-member AIDWA delegation to the NGO forum at Beijing. She was elected National President of AIDWA and to the Central Committee of the CPI(M) and to the Polit Bureau of the CPI(M).

Margaret Alva: lawyer, politician, parliamentarian, gender rights, activist she has served four consecutive terms of six years each, in the Rajya Sabha, in addition to one term in the Lok Sabha. During her 30 years in Parliament, she served on numerous important and prestigious committees, and chaired the Parliamentary Committee on the Empowerment of Woman. She was a Union Minister for 10 years, and served as Advisor to the Bureau of Parliamentary Studies and Training, as well as General Secretary of the All India Congress Committee. She was Governor of Uttarakhand, Rajasthan, Goa, and Gujarat. She is the founder president of Karuna, an NGO championing the cause of women, and children and has been active in the Women's Movement for over five decades. She is recipient of several awards in India and abroad including the First Nelson Mandela Award for Minority Empowerment in New York, The Shiromani Award for her contribution to Public Life, the Global Leadership Award from Vital Voices, Washington, and the Kannada Rajyothsava award.

Sunderlal Bahuguna: Gandhian peace worker, environmentalist and eco activist, has been one of the leaders of the Chipko movement, fighting for the preservation of forests in the Himalayas. In 1981 to 1983 he led a 5000 kilometer march across the Himalayas ending with a meeting with Indian Prime Minister Indira Gandhi, who then passed legislation to protect some areas of the Himalayan forests from clear-cutting. Sunderlal Bahuguna was also a leader in the movement to oppose the Tehri dam project and in defending India's rivers, and has also worked for women's rights and rights of the poor. In the tradition of Mahatma Gandhi, his work for change has always been done through peaceful resistance and other non-violent methods., He has co authored several book on preservation of the environment including *India's Environment: Myth & Reality* and *Environmental Crisis and Humans at Risk: Priorities for Action*. The Chipko Movement has received the 1987 Right Livelihood Award, also referred to as the Alternative Nobel Prize He was also awarded the Padma Shriand Padma Vibhushan and Jamnalal Bajaj Award for constructive work.

Murlidhar C. Bhandare: lawyer, human rights activist, writer, parliamentarian and politician, was a Professor of Law in Government Law College, Mumbai and was elected President of the Supreme Court Bar Association. He was elected to the Rajya Sabha thrice and was the Chairperson of the UN Sub-Commission on Prevention of Discrimination and Protection of Minorities, and was elected its Chairman. He was a Special Rapporteur of the UN Sub-Commission on the problems of Inter-relationship between international peace and effective materialization of all human rights, was a member of the Jury for the UN Human Rights Award, and a member of the UN Commission on Human Rights. He also had the opportunity to address the UN General Assembly and the first session of the UN Human Rights Council, Geneva in 2006. He was also the Governor of Odisha. Currently he is the managing trustee of the Justice Sunanda Bhandare Foundation, a leading NGO working towards ensuring gender equality, gender justice and empowerment of women. He has edited two volumes—T*he World of Gender Justice* and *Struggle for Gender Justice.*

Kamla Bhasin: gender rights activist, feminist, poet, writer, speaker, teacher, and institution builder, has been actively engaged with issues related to development, gender, men and masculinities, sustainable livelihoods, peace, identity politics, militarization, human rights education, media for the last five decades. She worked with the Food and Agriculture Organization of the United Nations. Currently, she works with Sangat, a Feminist Network, as Adviser, as well as JAGORI, a Women's Resource and Training Centre and Jagori Rural Charitable Trust as an active member. She is the South Asia Coordinator of One Billion Rising, a global campaign to end violence against women and girls and

Co-Chair of the worldwide network *Peace Women Across the Globe*; and member of South Asians for Human Rights (SAHR). Her main work at the South Asian level has included the capacity building of South Asian young activists and networking amongst civil society. She has also been conducting gender sensitisation workshops for senior non-governmental organization leaders and managers, government officials, police personnel, and members of Parliament in various countries of South Asia. She has written a large number of songs many of which have become anthems for the women's movement.

Dr. Lalit Bhasin: in legal practice for nearly six decades, was the Immediate Past President, The Bar Association of India, National Vice President, Indo-American Chambers of Commerce, president, Society of Indian Law Firms, Chairman, Chartered Institute of Arbitrators – India, President, Indian Law Foundation. He was also Former Chairman, Delhi Bar Council and the Film Certification Appellate Tribunal and former Member, International Court of Arbitration, paris, and was the Past President, Inter Pacific Bar Association. He was awarded the Plaque of Honour by the Prime Minister of India in 2002 for outstanding contributions to the Rule of Law and in n 2007, the President of India presented the National Law Day Award to him.

Ela R. Bhatt: a Gandhian, gender rights activist, institution builder, is widely recognized as one of the world's most remarkable pioneers and entrepreneurial forces in grassroots development. She founded the Self-Employed Women's Association (SEWA), a trade union with around 2 million members, the SEWA Cooperative Bank which has an outreach of 3 million women now. She was a nominated Member of the Rajya Sabha and subsequently Member of the Indian Planning Commission. She founded and served as Chair for Women's World Banking, the International Alliance of Home-based Workers, Street Vendors and Women in Informal Employment, Globalizing, Organizing, and as a trustee of the Rockefeller Foundation. She is the Chancellor of Gujarat Vidyapith University, founded by Mahatma Gandhi. She has received several awards, including Padmashree, Padmabhushan, the Ramon Magsaysay Award and the Right Livelihood Award, George Meany-Lane Kirkland Labour Rights Award by AFL-CIO, US, Indira Gandhi International Prize for Peace, Disarmament and Development, The Freedom from Want Medal' by Roosevelt Institute of the Netherlands. She has received honorary Doctorates from Harvard, Yale, Natal, McMaster, M. S. Baroda, and other Universities. She has written many books including *We Are Poor but So Many*.

Tara Gandhi Bhattacharjee: Gandhian, passionate exponent of non-violence, is the granddaughter of Mahtama Gandhi and C Rajagopalachari. She was Vice Chairperson of the Gandhi Smriti and Darshan Samiti, Birla house where, as a young teenager, she spent with him the last four months of the Mahatma's life. She is also involved with the movement to protect rivers, particularly the Save the Ganga movement for the last eighteen years. She has spent nearly three decades working with the Kasturba Gandhi National Memorial Trust, founded by the Mahatma as a civil society organization to serve the needy women and children of rural India. She has written *Reflections of an Extraordinary Era*, a behind-the-scenes biography of the Gandhi family and the tumult of India's independence. She was conferred the Officier de l'Ordre des Arts et Lettres by the French Government.

Zarina Bhatty: describes herself as humanist by faith, sociologist by profession and feminist by conviction. She has taught Sociology at Jesus and Mary college, University of Delhi, and was the President of Indian Association for Women's Studies (IAWS) and of Young Women's Christian Association (YWCA), New Delhi She has researched, published, and lectured extensively in India and abroad on Indian Muslim Women's issues and on women in the unorganized sector. Her pioneering study on women in the beedi industry, undertaken and published by the International Labour Organization (ILO), received considerable recognition She worked as Gender Specialist with United States Agency for International Development (USAID), International Fund for Agricultural Development (IFAD), and Islamic Development Bank (IDB). Her latest publication *Purdah to Piccadilly* which chronicles her experiences and struggles of breaking the stereotypes makes a compelling read. She is a recipient of the Devi Award.

Major General (Retd.) Ian Cardozo: writer, speaker and vociferous advocate of the rights of those disabled in war, was commissioned into the 1st Battalion the 5th Gorkha Rifles (Frontier Force) and was first officer of the Indian Army to be awarded the Sena Medal for gallantry on a patrol in North-Eastern Frontier He took part in the Sino-Indian war of 1962, the Indo-Pak war of 1965 and the Indo-Pak war of 1971. Wounded in the battle of Sylhet in Bangladesh, he overcame the disability of losing a leg and became the first disabled officer of the Indian Army to be approved for command of an infantry battalion and brigade. Thereafter, he commanded an Infantry Division and retired from this appointment as Chief of Staff of a Corps in the North-East. On retirement, he became the Chairman of the Rehabilitation Council of India and continued his work with the war disabled. Among his many books are *Param Vir, The Sinking of INS Khukri, The Bravest of the Brave– the Indian VCs of World War I*. He is also working with an illustrator in the area of graphic novels on the courage, competence and sacrifice of the Indian soldier, of which ten have been published so far.

Dr. Jyotsna Chatterjee: academician, and gender rights activist, is the Founder Director and Secretary of the Joint Women's Programme She was a Gender Trainer for the National Institute of Public Cooperation and Child Development, National Institute for Professional Advancement, Haryana Institute of

Public Administration, National Institute of Criminology, Police Training Centres and is the Governing Body Member of several organisations. She is the editor & author of several books & papers on women and children. During the course of her career, she convinced the Indian Government to make amendments to *Section 10 of the Indian Divorce Act, 1869*, which made divorce possible for both Christian men and women on equal grounds and divorce by mutual consent and was the driving force behind the passage of Devadasi Prohibition of Dedication Act against religious sanction for Child Prostitution through her study on the Devadasi Problem, and Trafficking of Women and Children. Her 10 workshops on Child Marriage in different regions of India sponsored by UNICEF and NHRC prepared the data for the passage of the new Act, *The Prohibition of Child Marriage Act.* She has received several awards including the Women of the Year Award from National Commission for Women, Women Achievers' Award from Amity University.

Mathew Cherian is the Chairperson of CARE India, is a member of the National Council of Senior Citizens chaired by the Prime Minister, and serves on the international board of HelpAge International. Earlier, he was a Member of the NGO Task Force of the Planning Commission, Member of the Grants Approval Committee of the Ministry of Social Justice & Empowerment, Member of Core Committee of National Human Rights Commission, and worked in the area of rural development with cooperatives in association with the National Dairy Development Board. He has also been: a consultant to voluntary agencies and to the National Wastelands Development Board; National Director, Oxfam, UK and India; Programme Director, South Asia, Plan International; Chief Executive Officer of HelpAge India; and Executive Director of the Charities Aid Foundation.

Dr. Shayama Chona: educationist, writer speaker, administrator and adocate for the rights of the differently abled, was Principal of Delhi Public School RK Puram, New Delhi, where she made successful efforts to break the barriers of schools to include the poor and the handicapped. Dr. Chona served as a member of over 99 Advisory Boards, Committees, Educational Institutions and is a member of UNESCO, and has has been associated with the Special Olympics, with Concerned Action Now and with the Society for Human Development. Working for upliftment of children suffering from multiple-handicapped, she has set up 3 centres for the mentally challenged: Tamana Special Centre, Tamana Nai Disha: Skill Development Centre, and the Tamana Autism Centre. She is the proud recipient of over 65 awards, the most prestigious being the Padma Shri, the Padma Bhushan, two other National Awards in 1997, and two State Awards for her investment in the field of education and social welfare.

Aruna Dalmia: philanthropist and social activist, is the founder and chairperson of Akshya Pratisthan, a voluntary organization working for the rehabilitation of the people with and without disability. Akshya Pratisthan is running a school of an integrated group of 410 children studying together in equal numbers from Nursery to Class VIII. Vocational training, sports & cultural activities are a part of the curriculum. She launched a Hydraulically Operated Tail Lift Bus for Persons With Disabilities, This was the First Tail Lift Bus in Asia and it earned the National Award from the Ministry of Woman and Child Development, Government of India. She and her organization have won many awards, including: the National Award for the Best Institute for Rehabilitation, from the Ministry of Social Justice & Empowerment; Bharat Nirman Award; Priyadarshini Award; and Manav Sewa Award.

Asha Das: bureaucrat, social activist, writer and speaker, joined the Indian Administrative Service in 1964 and was allotted to Madhya Pradesh state where among the many vital posts she held, she was Secretary of Revenue; Relief Commissioner; and Secretary of the Food and Civil Supplies and Cooperative Department.

Assignments in the Social Welfare and Women Development Departments gave her the opportunity to introduce distribution of hot cooked food to children at the Anganwadi Centres under the ICDS programme and encourage women's self-help groups to take on the task. During her tenures as Joint Secrteary and Secretary in the Ministry of Social Justice and Empowerment, and then as Secretary, Women and Child Development, in Delhi, she spearheaded the preparation and finalization of the Juvenile Justice Act, formulated guidelines for adoption of children in the country and abroad, evolved the Drug Abuse Prevention Progamme with comprehensive inter-disciplinary schemes for Counselling, Care and Treatment, and After care of Drug addicts. Under her, the Childline Foundation was set up to provide care and protection for Street Children; and the National Policy for the Aged was formulated.

Dr. Armaity S. Desai: social scientist, academician, professor, writer, and prolific speaker, was the Chairperson of the University Grants Commission, one of the only two women chairs. She was also Director at the prestigious Tata Institute of Social Sciences, which was also her alma mater She was also Principal of the College of Social Work. She taught in Chicago, from where she obtained her doctorate. She has been an active member of several national and international boards, and is currently Trustee, J. R. D. and Thelma Tata Trust; Member of the Advisory Committee, Campaign Against Child Labour; and Trustee, Childline Trust. She has been awarded The Katherine Kendall Distinguished Service Award for outstanding contribution to Social Work Education, by the International Association of Schools of Social Work (IASSW), USA, and the Professional Achievement Citation of the University of Chicago Alumni Association (1993).

Dr. A. B. Dey: doctor gerontologist, researcher, writer and professor, was the Founder Professor and Head of the

Department of Geriatric Medicine at the All India Institue of Medical Sciences, New Delhi. Ageing and Health care of older people being his primary area of interest, he has been trained in the International Institute on Ageing (UN-Malta). He has written over ten books and manuals and more than 150 articles. He is the Founder President of the Indian Academy of Geriatrics and his extensive research on ageing has resulted in establishing Geriatric Medicine as a sub-speciality of Medicine in India, and of the Development of National Programme for Health Care of older people. He has been awarded the "Vayoshrestha Samman" for the Department of Geriatric Medicine from the Ministry of Social Justice & Empowerment, Government of India, for contributions in research in Geriatrics. Currently he is providing assistance to the South-East Asia Regional Office of the World Health Organization in implementing its Healthy Ageing programs.

Dr. V. Mohini Giri: gender rights activist, peace advocate, writer, speaker and institution builder, was leader for four decades of the women's movement and specializes in human rights, gender justice and peace in India and South Asia. She represents and takes initiative for India's widows, a unique constituency. She is the founder chairperson of the War Widows Association, the Guild of Service and Women's Initiative for Peace in South Asia, governing body member of Foundation for Academic Access and Excellence, and the South Asian Network for Widows' Empowered in Development, was the Chairperson of National Commission for Women, trustee of the Gandhi Smriti and Darshan Samiti and Rajiv Gandhi Foundation, global director of the Hunger Project, and chairperson of the Review Committee for Policy on Older persons. She has been awarded extensively, including the Padma Bhushan Lifetime Achievement Award for building a society for All Ages by the NGO Committee on Ageing, United Nations; the Rajiv Gandhi Shiromani Award, and was nominated for Alternate Nobel Peace Prize among 1000 women peace activists across the globe.

Shivangi Gupta did her master's thesis on '*Sustaining the Sugarcane Value Chain in India*' which aimed to ensure environmental sustainability of biofuels produced as a sugar co-product in India. Currently working with Ms. Devaki Jain as a Research Assistant, Ms Gupta has been a Research Consultant to several organizations. She blogs on the development sector.

Dr. Syeda Hameed: feminist, gender rights activist, poet and writer and translator, is widely recognized for her passionate engagement in public affairs and social issues, especially for women, minorities, and peace. She is the Founder Member of the Muslim Women's Forum and a Founder Trustee of the Women's Initiative for Peace in South Asia. She was the Member of the Planning Commission of India, and Member of the National Commission for Women. A prolific writer she has authored and edited over 16 books including *Born to Be Hanged: Political Biography of Zulfikar Ali Bhutto, Gold Dust of Begum Sultans, Shahkar-e Adab, Bread, Beauty, Revolution: Khwaja Ahmad Abbas, K. G. Saiyidain: A Life in Education; Maulana Azad, Islam and the Indian National Movement, Beautiful Country: Stories from Another India*. She has been awarded the Padma Shri, Al-Ameen All India Community Leadership Award, Bi Amma Award, 2012 and Delhi Women of the Decade Achievers Award – Excellence in Governance.

Devaki Jain: economist, gender rights activist, writer and speaker and researcher, is an Honorary Fellow of St Anne's College, University of Oxford, from where she graduated. She was a lecturer in Economics in Delhi University but moved from teaching to full time research and publication as the director of the Institute of Social Studies Trust. Over the course of her career, she founded the Development Alternatives for Women for a new era (DAWN) – a third world network of women social scientists; and Institute of Social Studies Trust (ISST) – a research centre in Delhi. She has been a visiting fellow at Harvard University, Boston University, University of Sussex, SIAS, and Oxford University and has published more than 10 books as well as more than 100 papers related to 'Development with Women'. She was awarded the Padma Bhushan by the President of India in the Honours List of 2006, and an honorary doctorate from the University of Westville, Durban, South Africa.

Shanno Khurana: vocalist, musicologist and research scholar, a supreme exponent of the Rampur Gharana. Excels in the entire gamut of Hindustani musical forms and has performed in India, United States, London, Vienna, and Paris, through the Middle East, Southeast Asia and Tokyo in some of the most memorable performances of our times. She has produced substantial pieces of research on musicology, including the stylistic analysis and history of the eight major Hindustani *Gharanas*, and an in-depth musicological analysis and documentation of the folk music of Rajasthan. She composed, directed, and sang five operas. Troubled by the lot of women musicians, she started a festival called Bhairav-Se-Sohni in 1983 which has now grown into a nation-wide movement and has given a platform to Carnatic and Hindustani women-musicians who may not come from families of musicians and yet have been trained in the guru-shishya parampara. She was given the honorific of "Oltin Bulbule", the Golden Nightingale of the East, by UNESCO, and was awarded Padmashri, Padmabhushan, Panjabi Akademi Award, the Indira Gandhi Priyadarshani Award, Baba Alauddin Khan Award, amongst many others.

Rajni Kumar: teacher, educationist, and peace activist, has worked for more than sixty years in the field of education in India. She started her own school, Springdales School, as a kindergarten in the living room of her house, which has over the years, grown to four schools in India and one in Dubai and is reported to have had over 6000 students on its rolls. She was the chairperson of the Lady Irwin College and vice president of National Bal Bhavan. She has taken part in the Global Peace Conferences in Geneva, and the World Congress for the Rights of Children in Moscow. She is currently the Chairperson of Springdales Education Society, and also associated with the Delhi Schools Literacy Project, an initiative under the National Literacy Mission.. She has received a number of national and international recognitions for her work, including the Padma Shri, the "gr8! Women Award", and the Order of the Companions of O. R. Tambo (Silver) from the Government of South Africa.

Tahir Mahmood: legal scholar, academician, teacher, author and editor, served as the Dean of the Faculty of Law in Delhi University, chairman of Government of India's National Commission for Minorities, and Member of the Law Commission of India. Currently, he is with Amity University where his designation is Distinguished Jurist Chair, Professor of Eminence & Chairman, Institute of Advanced Legal Studies. He is on the Advisory Board of the Center for Law and Religion Studies at Brigham Young University (US), and the Steering Committee of the International Consortium of Law and Religion Studies at the University of Milan His major interest areas have been religion-state relations, Islamic law, and Indian family laws. He has authored over twenty books including *Laws of India on Religion and Religious Affairs, Religion; Law and Society across the Globe, Principles of Hindu Law: Personal Law of Hindus, Buddhists, Jains and Sikhs* and *Reminiscing on Law Brains: Bench, Bar and Academia*. He launched two prestigious journals – the *Islamic and Comparative Law Quarterly in 1981* and the *Religion and Law Review*. He has been awarded Shah Waliullah Award for Contemporary Understanding of Islamic Law and Distinguished Academic Services Award (USA).

Justice Sujata Manohar (Retd.): lawyer feminist and human rights activist and judge, was elevated as the first woman judge of the Bombay High Court and went on to become the Chief Justice of the Bombay High Court and thereafter of the Kerala High Court. She was the first woman Chief Justice of both the High Courts and was later on appointed as Judge of the Supreme Court of India. She was appointed Member, National Human Rights Commission, and was its Focal Point on Trafficking and Women's issues as well as on HIV/AIDS. She was Chairperson of the Committee on Feminism and International Law of the International Law Association and Consultant to the U. N. (DAW) expert group on Trafficking and to UN expert group on Women, Peace and Security. She is currently an arbitrator in national and international disputes. Among the many honours given to her are the National Law Day Award for Administration of Justice and the Capital Foundation Anil Divan National Award in Constitutional Law. She is Honorary Bencher of Lincoln's Inn, London, the first Indian judge to be so honoured, and holds Honorary Doctorates from various universities in India, US and U. K.

Dr. Raghunath Mashelkar: engineer, scientist research scholar and professor, has been the Director General of Council of Scientific and Industrial Research, Chairman of the National Innovation Foundation. He was also the President of the Indian National Science Academy, Global Research Alliance and Institute of Chemical Engineers (UK) and member of the Scientific Advisory Council to the Prime Minister In recognition of his pioneering research contributions in polymer science & Engineering, he has been honoured as a Fellow of Royal Society, Foreign Fellow of US National Academy of Sciences, among many other honours and conferred doctorates. He has more than 60 awards to his credit including the prestigious TWAS-Lenovo Science Prize, Business Week (USA) and the Padmashri, Padmabhushan, and the Padma Vibhushan.

Dr. George Mathew: sociologist, researcher Fulbright scholar, gender rights activist, social activist, writer and speaker is the Founder Director, Institute of Social Sciences, New Delhi His areas of specialisation are: local governance, grassroots democracy, the democratic process in India, decentralisation, gender equity and human rights. A prolific writer, he has participated and presented papers in international conferences on political process and democracy, religion and society and human rights. Dr. Mathew has served on various committees and commissions constituted by Government of India, State Governments, and International organisations. He was a visiting fellow at the South Asian Studies Centre, University of Chicago, and visiting Professor, University of Padova, and Universita Politecnica Delle Marche, Ancona, Italy; Shastri Indo-Canadian Institute Faculty Research Programme Fellowship, Trent University. Based on a true story, Dr. George Mathew produced the film: *Swaraaj: The Little Republic* which won the Gold Medal for the Best Film on Social Issues (2002) from the President of India for its strong depiction of women's empowerment in rural India.

Dr. Shovana Narayan: dancer, choreographer, research scholar, teacher writer, educationist and bureaucrat, has pursued two parallel exacting professional careers, achieving distinction and great heights in both. She is an acclaimed exponent as well as a guru of Kathak and has served in the Indian Audit and Accounts institutions till her retirement. She has written over 16 books, several research papers and well over 300 articles. She has been decorated by the Government of India with the Padmashri award, sangeet Natak Akademi award in 2001, and Delhi Government's Parishad Samman, besides being a recipient of 37 national and international awards. She is acknowledged as a classical example of a true Kathak, multi-faceted and dynamic, presenting a challenge to today's spectator.

Fali Sam Nariman: advocate, constitutional expert, professor, writer and speaker, is a Senior Advocate of the Supreme Court of India. He served as the Additional Solicitor–General of India and has been The President of the Bar Association of India, Vice–Chairman of the International Court of Arbitration of the International Chamber of Commerce, Paris, Member of the London Court of International Arbitration among many other prestigious positions held. He is a Visiting Professor of the National Law School of India University, Bangalore and was nominated as a member of the Rajya Sabha. Among his many books are *India's Legal System: Can It Be Saved?* and *Before Memory Fades... An Autobiography*. Awarded extensively, he is recipient of the Padma Bhushan, the Lal Bahadur Shastri Award for Excellence in Public Administration, Global Media Laurel at the International Conference of World Association of Press Councils, and the Justice Prize 2002 by the Peter Gruber Foundation and has been Named by the International Bar Association Headquarters in London as a "Living Legend of the Law".

Pascal Alan Nazareth: diplomat, writer and speaker, has served in India's diplomatic missions in Tokyo, Rangoon, Lima, London, New York, was Director General of the Indian Council for Cultural Relations (ICCR) and India's High Commissioner to Ghana and Ambassador to Egypt & Mexico. Since his retirement in May, 1994, he has lectured at numerous prestigious universities and Institutes in India and abroad, including the National Institute of Advanced Studies Bangalore, Benares Hindu University and Stanford, Yale, Columbia, Heidelberg, Uppsala & Peking Universities. His book *Gandhi's Outstanding Leadership* has come out in 12 Indian and 23 foreign languages. He was awarded the U Thant Peace Award for his 'Lifetime of World Service", and had the privilege of delivering the keynote addresses at the International day of Non Violence at the United Nations in New York and the United Nations Library in Geneva.

Lt. General (Retd.) Vijay Oberoi: was commissioned in 1 Maratha Li (Jangi Paltan) and participated in two wars: in Dec

1961, in capturing the Portuguese colony of Daman; and in the 1965 Indo-Pak War. It was in the latter that he had lost his right leg. Despite his disability, he soldiered on, till he retired as the Vice Chief of Army Staff. His command appointments include command of an armoured division, a strike corps and two Commands - Army Training Command and Western Command; his staff appointments include heading the Perspective Planning Directorate, before being appointed DGMO. He was an International Fellow at the United States Army War College, and Defence Adviser of India in Malaysia. A prolific writer, he has edited five books and contributed chapters in many others. He was the Founder Director of the Centre for Land Warfare Studies (CLAWS) for five years. He is currently the Founder President of the War Wounded Foundation, set up for meaningful rehabilitation of war disabled personnel. He is the recipient of all three distinguished service awards: Vishisht Sewa Medal, Ati Vishisht Sewa Medal and the Param Vishisht Sewa Medal.

Lt. General (Retd.) Shankar Prasad: was commissioned into the elite 3 Gorkha Rifles Since then, he has served in various command and staff appointments of the Indian Army including Command of an Infantry Brigade with Indian Peace Keeping Force (IPKF) in Sri Lanka, Command of National Anti Hijack Force of the Commandos of the National Security Guards (NSG), and Command of a Pivot Corps on the Western borders with Pakistan; Deputy Director General in the Military Operations Directorate in the Army Head Quarters; Inspector General of the Army at the Army Headquarters. Post retirement, he is a Defence Analyst for various domestic and foreign TV and Radio channels including the BBC, covering issues concerning national security, diplomacy, terrorism, and related matters, and has contributed to the development of policies of national disaster management, particularly in the field of NBC terrorism. He has written two books, *The Gallant Dogras* and *The Infantry*. He has been awarded the Vishisht Sewa Medal, and the ParamVishisht Sewa Medal.

Arun Bharat Ram: industrialist, philanthropist, sitar artist, Chairman of SRF Limited, is credited with turning his family-owned multi-business organization into a world class conglomerate. Today, SRF's business portfolio covers Fluorochemicals, Specialty Chemicals, Packaging Films, Technical Textiles, Coated and Laminated Fabrics, across eleven manufacturing plants in India, and one each in Thailand, South Africa, and Hungary. He serves as the chairman of SRF Foundation, which runs one of the largest community programs in the country, imparting education and vocational training programs to underprivileged children and youth by improving the infrastructure facilities in Government schools, promoting computer-aided learning, and through the digital inclusion of communities. Among his many talents, he is also an accomplished sitar player.

Lalita Ramdas: teacher, feminist, human rights activist, says that inner awakening as a person evolves through a process of Education to Reality – deeply influenced by Liberation Theology – Marxist analysis – Freire, Lao Tsu, Tagore– and personal praxis, She believes the Personal is Political and has tried to integrate the political in the personal She revels in the challenge of straddling, reconciling, transforming and recreating the many identities, roles, and worlds she has inhabited through her 80 years and chooses to call her self a Subversive Educator at Large. In the early 1980s, she put in place pathbreaking initiatives for development education in a number of elite schools. She was president of the International Council for Adult Education and founded Ankur, a society for alternatives in education. She has worked for years as a simple community-level non-formal educator in Delhi's slums, participated in street theatre to raise awareness of dowry, rape, and other gender issues. Currently living in a small village in India's west coast, she is involved in the life of the local community while pursuing citizens' peace initiatives with Pakistan and contributing to the global adult education movement.

Ashok Sajjanhar: diplomat, writer speaker, communal harmony activist; was ambassador of India to Kazakhstan, Sweden and Latvia and has worked in senior diplomatic positions in Indian Embassies/Missions in Washington DC, Brussels, Moscow, Geneva, Tehran, Dhaka and Bangkok, and also at Headquarters in India. He negotiated for India in the Uruguay Round of Multilateral Trade Negotiations and in negotiations for India-EU, India-ASEAN and India-Thailand Free Trade Agreements. He worked as head of the National Foundation for Communal Harmony to promote amity and understanding between different religions, faiths, and beliefs. He has been decorated by Governments of Kazakhstan and Latvia with their National Awards and by Universal Peace Federation, New York with Title of "Ambassador of Peace." He is currently President of Institute of Global Studies, and Distinguished Fellow, Ananta Aspen Centre, New Delhi.

As the daughter of a freedom fighter, **Padma Seth** had her leadership skills honed in childhood itself. A lawyer by training, she is a dynamic social activist with an abiding interest in the issues of women and children. She served as Director of the National Bal Bhawan for twelve years, and was a very active member of the National Commission for Women. Her books include the acclaimed *Infant Mortality and Maternal Mortality*.

Sushma Seth: versatile actress, teacher of speech and drama, and a children's theatre activist, has played lead roles in over 80 plays, in Hindi, Urdu and English theatre in an eminently successful career spanning six decades. She has directed over 40 plays She has also acted in over a 100 films and television series. Notable among them were *Hum Log* and *Dekh Bhai Dekh*. She is a Founder Member of Yatrik, and established Children's Creative Theatre, and initiated the Childrens' drama workshops at the National School of Drama. Currently she is the Honorary Cultural Director of an inter-faith NGO Arpana. Among her many awards are the Rashtriya Priyadarshini Award, Bharat Nirman Award, Best Actress Award from Sahitya Kala Parishad, Kalpana Chawla Excellence Award, Sangeet Natak Akademi Tagore Award for her contribution toIndian theatre, and the National Vayoshreshtha Samman from the Ministry of Social Justice and Empowerment for Creative Arts.

Dr. Mala Kapur Shankardass: sociologist, gerontologist, health and development social scientist, works as Associate Professor at Maitreyi College, University of Delhi. She has also been Consultant with the World Health Organization, SEARO and with the International Institute on Ageing, Malta. She is the Asia Representative of the International Network for Prevention of Elder Abuse, managing trustee of Development, Welfare and Research Foundation and governing body member of the Alzheimer's and Related Disorders Society of India, She writes extensively on ageing, including *Growing Old in India: Voices Reveal, Statistics Speak*, and has edited many books including *Abuse and Neglect of the Elderly in India, International Handbook of Elder Abuse and Mistreatment, Combatting Elder Abuse in Australia and India.* She is also author of Monographs commissioned by the United Nations. She is Editorial Board Member, *Journal of Adult Protection, Polish Social Gerontology Journal*, and Member of the National Advisory Board of the *Journal of the Indian Academy of Geriatrics*, and Member of the Advisory Board of the *Journal of Mental Health.*

Dr. V. Shanta: doctor, cancer specialist, the Chairman & Executive Chairman of the Cancer Institute (WIA) Chennai, a major comprehensive Cancer Centre of national and international stature, has dedicated over 50 years of her life to the mission of organising care of Cancer patients, the study of the disease, its prevention and control, and the generation of specialists and scientists in different aspects of Oncologic Sciences. She was member of the WHO Advisory Committee on Cancer, Chairman of the INDO-US Collaborative Group on Lymphoid Neoplasias (Indian Chapter), President of the Asian & Pacific Federation of Organisations for cancer control, and Member, Kudankulam Nuclear Power Project. Among her many awards, she is a recipient of the Padma Shri, Padma Bhushan and Padma Vibushan, and the Ramon Magsaysay Award for Public Service.

Dr. Urmil Sharma: gynaecologist, writer, teacher speaker and social activist, has served as a Consultant in Lok Nayak Jaiprakash Narayan Hospital and the prestigious All India Institute of Medical Sciences and was actively involved in teaching and clinical practice. She has been awarded the Fellowship of the Royal College of Gynaecologists (FRCOG) and was a WHO consultant for providing expert care in Gynaecological surgery in countries of the South-East Asia Region. She was President of the Indian Medical Association, Delhi, and has been lecturing for the last two decades in various social organisations, the UN, and WHO. She has been very active in social activities related to the medical profession.

General (Retd.) V. N. Sharma: PVSM, AVSM, retired as the Chief of the Army Staff (COAS), after 40 years' distinguished commissioned service. As an Army Commander, the General commanded India's Eastern Army where he aggressively managed the India-China high-altitude borders against offensive infiltrating Chinese patrols. During his tenure as army chief, he successfully completed the operations of the Indian Peace Keeping Force (IPKF) in Sri Lanka. He masterminded the Indian tri-service swift operational landing operations in the Maldives when President Gayoom's government had been overtaken by insurgent groups from northern Sri Lanka, and Maldives. He commenced the destruction, of serious insurgent and terrorist groups trained and armed by Pakistan, in Punjab and J&K in 1989-90 and effectively neutralized them. He is a trustee of Cheshire Homes, Delhi, a charity NGO looking after paraplegics, and he is Chairman of an Educational Trust created by the alumni of the Rashtriya Indian Military College. He also personally contributes to and runs a free medical clinic in village Dadh in Kangra District, Himachal Pradesh. He has been awarded the Ati Vishisht Sewa Medal and the ParamVishisht Sewa Medal.

Dr. Karan Singh: politician, philanthropist, writer and poet, is the son of Maharaja Hari Singh, was the Prince Regent of Jammu and Kashmir, and became successively President (Sadr-i-Riyasat) and Governor of the state. He worked closely with Jawaharlal Nehru, and with Sardar Patel during the founding of the Republic of India, and in 1967 became the youngest-ever union cabinet minister in the government of Indira Gandhi. He was a member of the Rajya Sabha, and senior member of the Indian National Congress Party, a life trustee and president of the India International Center, and was for three terms Chancellor of Banaras Hindu University . During the conclusion of the Cold War, he was India's ambassador to the USA. He is a recipient of the Padma Vibhushan.

Dr. Mohinder Singh: academician, teacher social activist and writer, has served as Director, Guru Nanak Foundation, as Member, National Commission for Minority Educational Institutions, as Professor of Eminence, Punjabi University, as Director, National Institute of Panjab Studies, and Bhai Vir Singh Sahitya Sadan and Visiting Professor of Sikhism, Centre for Global Studies, University of California. Currently he is Professor-Director, National Institute of Panjab Studies. Dr. Singh was awarded a Fellowship by the Indian Council of Historical Research to carry on his research work on the Akali Movement in the United Kingdom, which later earned him his Doctorate. Author of several standard works on Sikh history and religion,

Dr. Singh sits on the Advisory Boards of several national and international organisations.

Multi-talented **Sunanda Singhania** is a passionate gardener, and Executive Director of the Pushpawati Singhania Hospital & Research Institute in Delhi which is a result of the sense of social responsibility that her family advocates, affirms and lives by. The outreach to build social capital is not restricted to hospitals alone but extends to mobile dispensaries to serve villages, adult literacy classes and schools. She has given a professional dimension to her love for travelling as she also is the Executive Director of Uniglobe Indica Travels & Tours.

Zena Sorabjee: educationist and social activist, is Chairman of the Lotus Charitable Trust, and of the King George Memorial Committee, an institution providing shelter for the destitute in Mumbai. She is a Trustee of the Barli Development Institute for Rural Women in Indore, Madhya Pradesh. Additionally, she is the Vice Chairman of the Guild for Service, New Delhi, and the Vice Chairman of the National Spiritual Assembly of the Baha'is of India. Over the years, she has been supporting projects in rural education, the education of girls, and the transfer of technology to rural India. She started the Brilliant Stars School in Tripura to empower youth to become agents of positive socio-economic transformation in their communities. She authored the children's book *The Right to Be* which was a unique attempt to introduce children to the concept of human rights.

Dr. Uma Tuli: academician, educationist and social activist, she has consistently spearheaded the cause of disabled people. She is the founder of the Amar Jyoti Charitable Trust rendering rehabilitative services at Delhi and Gwalior with the holistic approach of providing integrated education, vocational training, medical care and self-employment within one campus.

She was Chief Commissioner for Persons with Disabilities, and an Executive Member of International Abilympics Federation, and Chairperson – Education Commission Rehabilitation International, USA. The Amar Jyoti Charitable Trust is the recipient of two National Awards - for the best institution in 1991, and for the creation of barrier free environment in 2005. Among the numerous awards for her dedicated work, she has received the Padma Shri, Helen Keller Award, UN-ESCAP appreciation, the Hong Kong Foundation Award, Nehru Smriti Award, Women Achievers award, Lakshmipat Singhania-IIM Lucknow National Leadership Award 2010, and President's Gold Medal for distinctive services in Home Guards.

Dr. Saroja Vaidyanathan: notable exponent of Bharatanatyam, choreographer, guru, writer and institution builder. She is the founder director of the Ganesa Natyalaya school for Bharta Natyam and Carnatic vocal music She is a prolific choreographer and has to her credit ten full length ballets, and nearly two thousand individual Bharatanatyam items. She undertook a cultural tour of South East Asia accompanying the then Prime Minister's visit to the ASEAN Summit. She has also published her renditions of Subramania Bharati's songs and poems and some of his works have also been set to dance by her. She has written a number of books on Bharatanatyam and Carnatic music, including *The Classical Dances of India, Bharatanatyam – An In-Depth Study, Carnataka Sangeetham*, and *The Science of Bharatanatyam*. Among her many awards are the Padma Shri, Padma Bhushan, Snageet Natak Akademi Award, Sahitya Kala Parishad Samman and she was conferred the title of 'Bharata Kalai Sudar'.

Aruna Vasudev: is an Indian critic, author, editor, painter, and maker of documentaries, and is considered an eminent scholar of Asian cinema. She has also been described as the mother of Asian Cinema. She is Founder and now President-Emeritus of the Network for the Promotion of Asia-Pacific

Cinema (NETPAC International), Founder-Editor of *Cinemaya* – The Asian Film Quarterly, Founder-Director of *Cinefan*, the Cinemaya Festival of Asian Cinema, and Founder-Director of *The Inner Path* Festival of Buddhist Film Art & Philosophy. She is an author and film critic with a PhD from the University of Paris. She is the author of two books on Indian cinema She has won a number of awards internationally for her work, including the Star of Italian Solidarity from Italy, the Officer of Arts & Letters from France, Lifetime Achievement awards from film festivals and organisations in Iran, Korea, Sri Lanka, Hawaii, Philippines, India, etc., and has been member, or president, of more than 40 international juries.

Padma Venkataraman: social activist, yoga enthusiast, musician, institution builder, and has been active in grassroots work in Socio economic rehabilitation of Leprosy-affected people for 25 years. She was the permanent representative of the All-India Women's Conference to the UN in Vienna, Vice President of International NGO committee on Women, President of United Nations Women's Guild, President of Gnanodaya Rehabilitation Association and Trustee, Global Cancer Concern India, among many other positions she has held. As the Honorary Director of All India Women's Conference-FAO (United Nations Food and Agriculture Organisation) partnership Project for leprosy patients in the 4000 strong Shahadara colony in Delhi she also worked with "Hope Worldwide" to construct homes for 800 families. She founded along with Werner Dornik, Austrian MultiMedia Artist, the Bindu Art Trust which has restored self confidence and self respect to leprosy-affected people through art. Among her many awards is the Hand on Hope from Hope World Wide – USA, the International Humanitarian Service Award by Mentor International, USA, Malala Award for best supporter of differenty-abled, and Award by the Universal Peace Foundation.

Kalpakam Yechury is committed gender rights activist, and Trustee of All India Women's Conference, which has a pan India presence with multiple branches, and is one of the oldest civil society organisations committed to the rights of underprivileged women and children. She was the first woman driver to participate in a car rally over the Himalayas.

Zakia Zaheer is an Urdu litterateur, author of *Zindagi Zinda Dilli Ka Naam Hai*, and translator into Urdu of William Dalrymple's *The Last Mughal* and of Qaisra Shahraz's *Holy Woman*. She was awarded the Indira Gandhi Priyadarshini Award in 2014.